WORKBOOK TO ACCOMPANY DELMAR'S

ADMINISTRATIVE MEDICAL ASSISTING

Fourth Edition

Gerry A. Brasin, AS, CMA (AAMA), CPC
Corporate Education Coordinator
Premier Education Group
Springfield, MA

Barbara M. Dahl, CMA (AAMA), CPC
Program Director
Whatcom Community College
Bellingham, WA

Comprehensive Examination by:
Tricia Berry, MATL, OTR/L
Assistant Dean of Clinical Placement
School of Health Sciences
Kaplan University
Johnston, IA

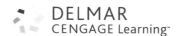

DELMAR
CENGAGE Learning·

Australia • Brazil • Japan • Mexico • Singapore • Spain • United Kingdom • United States

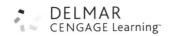

DELMAR
CENGAGE Learning

Workbook to Accompany Delmar's Administrative Medical Assisting, Fourth Edition
Gerry A. Brasin, Barbara M. Dahl, and Tricia Berry

Vice President, Career and Professional Editorial: Dave Garza

Director of Learning Solutions: Matthew Kane

Senior Acquisitions Editor: Rhonda Dearborn

Managing Editor: Marah Bellegarde

Senior Product Manager: Sarah Prime

Editorial Assistant: Chiara Astriab

Vice President, Career and Professional Marketing: Jennifer McAvey

Executive Marketing Manager: Wendy E. Mapstone

Senior Marketing Manager: Nancy Bradshaw

Marketing Coordinator: Erica Ropitzky

Production Director: Carolyn Miller

Content Project Manager: Anne Sherman

Senior Art Director: Jack Pendleton

Production Technology Analyst: Tom Stover

For product information and technology assistance, contact us at
Professional Group Cengage Learning Customer & Sales Support, 1-800-354-9706

For permission to use material from this text or product, submit all requests online at **www.cengage.com/permissions.**
Further permissions questions can be emailed to
permissionrequest@cengage.com.

Library of Congress Control Number: 2008930399

ISBN-13: 978-1-4354-1923-0

ISBN-10: 1-4354-1923-5

Delmar
5 Maxwell Drive
Clifton Park, NY 12065-2919
USA

Cengage Learning is a leading provider of customized learning solutions with office locations around the globe, including Singapore, the United Kingdom, Australia, Mexico, Brazil, and Japan. Locate your local office at: **international.cengage.com/region**

Cengage Learning products are represented in Canada by Nelson Education, Ltd.

To learn more about Delmar, visit **www.cengage.com/delmar**
Purchase any of our products at your local college store or at our preferred online store **www.ichapters.com**

For your lifelong learning solutions, visit **delmar.cengage.com**
Visit our corporate website at **www.cengage.com**

Printed in the United States of America
1 2 3 4 5 6 7 12 11 10 09

CONTENTS

This workbook is part of a dynamic learning system that will help reinforce the essential competencies you need to enter the field of medical assisting and become a successful, multiskilled medical assistant. It has been completely revised to challenge you to apply the chapter knowledge from *Delmar's Administrative Medical Assisting*, Fourth Edition, to develop basic competencies, use critical thinking skills, and integrate your knowledge effectively.

WORKBOOK ORGANIZATION

The Chapter Assignment Sheets are divided into the following sections: Chapter Pre-Test, Vocabulary Builder, Learning Review, Certification Review, Learning Application, Chapter Post-Test, and Self-Assessment. The content of the workbook has been designed to give you a creative and interpretive forum to apply the knowledge you have learned, not simply to repeat information to answer questions. Realistic simulations appear throughout the workbook that reference the characters in the textbook. This gives the material a real-world feel that comes as close as possible to your future experiences in an ambulatory setting. Clinical principles, such as infection control or communication and patient education, are repeatedly reinforced through simulation exercises that require the ability to use your knowledge effectively and readily.

COMPETENCY ASSESSMENT CHECKLISTS

Competency Assessment Checklists are designed to set criteria or standards that should be observed while a specific procedure is being performed. The procedural steps are listed in the textbook, and the Competency Assessment Checklist scoring reflects the major milestones, or outcomes, of following the specific procedural steps. As you perform each procedure, the evaluation section of this checklist can be used to judge your performance. The instructor will use this checklist to evaluate your competency in performing this skill. Your instructor may combine some Competencies and adjust others to suit individual program schedules. These checklists are provided for guidance.

A master Competency Assessment Tracking Sheet is also provided for you prior to this section of the workbook to use as an overview of all competency assessment checklists. This tracking sheet can serve as a table of contents for all checklists, as well as a guide to easily view your performance on the assessment checklists.

The format of the Competency Assessment Checklists is designed to provide specific conditions, standards, milestone steps, and evaluation and documentation sections for essential skills necessary for an entry-level medical assistant. Forms are provided on the Student Online Companion for use with the competency assessment checklists as you complete the procedures in your textbook. To access the Student Online Companion, use the instructions on the tear-out Access Card in your book to create your account and log in.

COMPREHENSIVE EXAMINATION

Feel certain that each procedure and concept you master is an important step toward preparing your skills and knowledge for the workplace. A final comprehensive examination is presented at the conclusion of the workbook, covering all the essential topic areas that medical assisting graduates must master. This examination has 200 questions and provides excellent practice for national certification examinations.

iv

FINAL THOUGHTS

The textbook, software CDs, workbook, and online companion have all been coordinated to meet the core objectives. Review the performance objectives at the beginning of each chapter in the textbook before you begin to study; they are a road map that will take you to your goals.

Remember that you are the learner, so you can take credit for your success. The instructor is an important guide on this journey, and the text, workbook, student software CD, and practicums are tools, but whether or not you use the tools wisely is ultimately up to you.

Evaluate yourself and your study habits. Take positive steps toward improving yourself, and avoid habits that could limit your success. Do family responsibilities and social opportunities interfere with your study? If so, sit down with your family and plan a schedule for study that they will support and to which you will adhere. Find a special place to study that is free from distraction.

Because regulations vary from state to state regarding which procedures can be performed by a medical assistant, it will be important to check specific regulations in your state. A medical assistant should never perform any procedure without being aware of legal responsibilities, correct procedure, and proper authorization.

As you pursue a wonderful career in medical assisting, make the most of your education and training.

Chapter Assignment Sheets

C H A P T E R **3**

History of Medicine

CHAPTER PRE-TEST

Perform this test without looking at your book. If an answer is "false," rewrite the sentence to make it true.

1. True or False? The practice of medicine began when we started keeping medical records.

_____

_____

2. True or False? Plants used to be the basis of all medications but are not anymore.

_____

_____

3. True or False? Cultural differences do not and should not influence the way we treat our patients.

_____

_____

4. True or False? Magic was practiced because it was considered an essential ingredient in chasing evil spirits away.

_____

_____

5. True or False? Ancient Eastern treatments included curing the spirit and nourishing the body.

_____

_____

6. True or False? Acupuncture uses the placement of needles in thousands of points on the body.

_____

_____

7. True or False? Women were not accepted as medical doctors in Western culture until the 1800s.

_____

_____

8. True or False? The "father of preventive medicine" was Louis Pasteur.

_____

_____

9. True or False? Edward Jenner developed the smallpox vaccine in the late 1700s.

_____

_____

10. True or False? The Oath of Hippocrates mentions mischief, sexual misconduct, and slaves.

_____

_____

VOCABULARY BUILDER

Misspelled Words

Find the words below that are misspelled; circle them, and correctly spell them in the spaces provided. Then insert the correct vocabulary terms from the list that best fit the descriptions below.

acepsis	malaria	septacemia
acupuncture	opiods	typhis
alopathic	pharmacopoies	yellow fever
bubonic plague	pluralistic	

_____   _____   _____

_____   _____   _____

1. In our _____ society, we rely on several philosophies of medicine that serve an individual's needs by respecting ethnic, cultural, and religious traditions while providing the best standard of care to patients and their families.

2. The piercing of the skin by long needles into any of 365 points along 12 meridians that traverse the body and transmit an active life force called qi is the practice of _____, an ancient Chinese technique thought by many today to be effective in the treatment of chronic pain.

3. That bacteria can enter the bloodstream to cause infection, _____, was observed in the nineteenth century by Hungarian physician and obstetrician Ignaz Philipp Semmelweiss.

4. Since the twentieth century, the discovery of antibiotics, the development of vaccines, and the institution of proper health and sanitation measures have largely contributed to the containment of many infectious diseases, including _____, _____, and _____.

5. _____ physicians treat illness and disease with medical and surgical interventions intended to alleviate the condition or effect a cure.

6. A _____ is a book that describes drugs and their preparation and details plant, animal, and mineral substances as essential ingredients in effecting cures.

7. In the nineteenth century, _____, the process of sterilizing surgical environments to discourage the growth of bacteria, and anesthesia, the process of alleviating pain during surgery, revolutionized surgical practices throughout the world.

LEARNING REVIEW

Short Answer

1. Religion, magic, and science all play a vital part in the history of medicine. Describe each.

   Religion _____

   _____

   Magic _____

   _____

   Science _____

   _____

   _____

2. Name the five methods of treatment important to the practice of medicine according to ancient Chinese tradition. How are these methods relevant for allopathic physicians today?

   _____

   _____

   _____

   _____

   _____

   _____

   _____

   _____

   _____

3. Individual cultures and people throughout history have conferred different, and often changing, status upon women in medicine. For each of the five cultures below, describe the status of women in medicine.

   (1) Primitive societies:

   _____

   _____

   (2) Chinese:

   _____

   (3) Muslim:

   _____

   (4) Italian:

   _____

   _____

(5) American:

_____

_____

4. Trace the progression of medical education by listing the important advances, discoveries, or medical philosophies for each period or century listed. What do you expect for the twenty-first century?

(1) Prehistoric times:

_____

_____

_____

(2) Ancient times:

_____

_____

_____

_____

_____

(3) Seventh century:

_____

_____

_____

_____

(4) Ninth century:

_____

_____

_____

(5) Renaissance:

_____

_____

_____

_____

(6) Nineteenth century:

_____

_____

_____

_____

(7) Twentieth century:

_____
_____
_____
_____
_____
_____

(8) Twenty-first century:

_____
_____

5. Attitudes toward illness have changed throughout the history of medicine and also often differ among cultures. For each situation listed, give both historical and current attitudes toward the sick person. Discuss how attitudes toward illness may, or may not, have changed through history.

(1) Elderly and infirm people are encouraged to end their own lives or are outcast from society.

_____
_____
_____
_____
_____

(2) Individuals with a frightening illness, for which there is no cure, are shunned or quarantined.

_____
_____
_____
_____
_____

(3) Sickness is seen as a moral or spiritual failing of an individual.

_____
_____
_____
_____
_____

(4) Survivors of illness are viewed as heroic individuals.

_____
_____
_____
_____

(5) People with disabilities are valued as individuals and receive care that allows them to function in mainstream society.

_____

_____

_____

_____

6. Name 15 infectious or epidemic diseases that have been controlled in the twentieth century through medical advances and discoveries such as antibiotics, vaccines, asepsis, and insulin.

_____

_____

_____

7. The Hippocratic Oath, which originated in ancient Greece, embodies within it many ethical standards of treatment and care that providers espouse to this day. In contemporary layperson's language, name the five basic standards contained in the oath.

_____

_____

_____

_____

_____

8. Fill in the blanks below with the three epidemics discussed in the chapter, along with descriptions of each and treatment options.

Epidemic   **Description, Causes, Treatment**

_____   _____

                               _____

                               _____

                               _____

_____   _____

                               _____

                               _____

                               _____

_____   _____

                               _____

                               _____

                               _____

Matching I

For each of the following, write an R if the statement describes a belief in religion, an M if the statement describes a belief in magic, or an S if the statement describes a belief in science.

_____ 1. A recent research study involved two groups of patients with AIDS: One group received daily prayers from an anonymous prayer group hundreds of miles away, and the other received no prayers. The group receiving the prayers responded better to treatment.

_____ 2. Trephination was used by prehistoric cultures to release evil spirits responsible for illness.

_____ 3. Chinese acupuncture techniques are used to control pain or treat drug dependency.

_____ 4. Botanicals are effective in treating certain conditions. The Chinese pharmacopoeia is rich in the use of herbs.

_____ 5. Some Native Americans believe that someone recovering from a serious illness might hold extraordinary powers.

_____ 6. Some practitioners throughout history have held to the belief that healing involves not just medical treatment, but attention to the purity of the patient's soul and to the faith of the individual as well.

Matching II

Match the individuals listed below with each of their contributions to the history of medicine.

_____	1. Andreas Vesalius	A. Developed a vaccine for poliomyelitis
_____	2. Sir Alexander Fleming	B. "Father of medicine"
_____	3. W. T. G. Morton	C. Developed smallpox vaccine
_____	4. Moses	D. Discovered penicillin
_____	5. Edward Jenner	E. "Father of bacteriology"
_____	6. Clara Barton	F. Advocate of health rules in Hebrew religion
_____	7. Louis Pasteur	G. Invented the stethoscope
_____	8. Elizabeth Blackwell	H. First female physician in the United States
_____	9. Hippocrates	I. Rendered accurate anatomical drawings of body systems
_____	10. René Laënnec	J. Wrote first anatomical studies
_____	11. Robert Koch	K. Laid the groundwork for asepsis
_____	12. Florence Nightingale	L. Started the American Red Cross
_____	13. Anton van Leeuwenhoek	M. Founder of modern nursing
_____	14. Wilhelm von Roentgen	N. Introduced ether as an anesthetic
_____	15. John Hunter	O. Discovered lens magnification
_____	16. Elizabeth G. Anderson	P. Discovered X-rays
_____	17. Leonardo da Vinci	Q. Founder of scientific surgery
_____	18. Joseph Lister	R. Developed culture-plate method
_____	19. Jonas Salk	S. Discovered insulin
_____	20. Frederick G. Banting	T. First female physician

CERTIFICATION REVIEW

These questions are designed to mimic the certification examination. Select the best response.

1. Who of the following was not a scientist who contributed to the study of bacteriology?

    a. Louis Pasteur

    b. Robert Koch

    c. Joseph Lister

    d. John Hunter

2. The first female physician in the United States was:

    a. Clara Barton

    b. Elizabeth Blackwell

    c. Florence Nightingale

    d. Joan of Arc

3. The Oath of Hippocrates:

    a. establishes guidelines for all health care providers

    b. establishes guidelines for the practice of medicine

    c. is a well-known document about the ethics of ancient medicine

    d. was the first scientific journal of significance

4. The ancient culture that believed that illness was a punishment by the gods for violations of moral codes was the:

    a. Chinese

    b. Egyptian

    c. Mesopotamian

    d. Indian

5. Ancient healing priests performed many functions that involved the welfare of the entire community or village and were referred to as:

    a. shamans

    b. chi

    c. lipuria

    d. polypenia

6. Medical education in established universities began in what century?

    a. Second

    b. Fifteenth

    c. Eighteenth

    d. Ninth

7. What country today quarantines everyone who tests positive for HIV, even if they show no signs of the disease?

   a. Africa

   b. Cuba

   c. Korea

   d. Canada

8. In 1922, insulin was established as a treatment for diabetes by:

   a. Lister

   b. Pasteur

   c. Salk and Sabin

   d. Banting and Best

LEARNING APPLICATION

 CASE STUDY

When 52-year-old Margaret Thomas, Martin Gordon's younger sister, begins to experience mild hand tremors and balance problems, Martin suggests that Margaret go see Dr. Winston Lewis. Dr. Lewis is Martin's primary care provider, who had provided treatment for Martin's prostate cancer. Feeling more comfortable with a female physician, Margaret chooses to make an appointment with Dr. Lewis's associate in the group practice, Dr. Elizabeth King. On the day of the examination, she brings her 25-year-old daughter with her to the clinic.

After taking a detailed patient history and undertaking a thorough physical examination of Margaret, Dr. King makes note of signs and symptoms, including a resting tremor, shuffling gait, muscle rigidity, and difficulty in swallowing and speaking. Margaret also complains of a "hot feeling" and odd, uncharacteristic moments of defective judgment when "she just can't keep things straight." Dr. King suspects Parkinson's disease and tells Margaret and her daughter that she would like to refer Margaret to a neurologist for more specific examination and medical tests. Dr. King explains that there are effective drug therapies for controlling the disease, although it has no known cure, and that the neurologist will outline Margaret's treatment options if a diagnosis of Parkinson's is made. Margaret seems to be shaken but takes Dr. King's words in stride.

Dr. King leaves Margaret and her daughter in the examination room with Audrey Jones, CMA (AAMA), who has assisted Dr. King throughout the examination and asks Audrey to be sure to give Margaret the referral to the neurologist. Margaret's daughter asks Audrey if Parkinson's is the disease that has shown promise in fetal tissue research and if her mother might be a candidate. Before Audrey can answer, Margaret becomes visibly distressed. "We're a good Catholic family, I could never consider that. Me—a grandmother." Looking to Audrey, she adds, "Please tell me I won't be involved with such a thing."

continues

CASE STUDY REVIEW QUESTIONS

1. What part does the role of women in medicine and in society play in this situation?

   _____

   _____

   _____

   _____

   _____

   _____

   _____

   _____

2. How should Audrey, the medical assistant, reply to Margaret and her daughter? What course of action, if any, should she take?

   _____

   _____

   _____

   _____

   _____

3. How do religious beliefs make an impact on the attitude toward illness held by the patient? How might these beliefs affect a treatment plan?

   _____

   _____

   _____

   _____

   _____

4. Discuss the issues that arise when a potential medical breakthrough involves controversial or radical ideas that challenge long-held cultural viewpoints and beliefs.

   _____

   _____

   _____

   _____

   _____

   _____

   _____

CHAPTER POST-TEST

Perform this test without looking at your book. If an answer is "false," rewrite the sentence to make it true.

1. True or False? The practice of medicine began long before we started keeping medical records.

   _____

   _____

2. True or False? Plants remain the basis of many medications.

   _____

   _____

3. True or False? Cultural differences do and should influence the way we treat our patients.

   _____

   _____

4. True or False? Magic has never played a role in medicine.

   _____

   _____

5. True or False? Ancient Eastern treatments did not include working with the human spirit.

   _____

   _____

6. True or False? Acupuncture uses the placement of needles in 365 points on the body.

   _____

   _____

7. True or False? Women were accepted as medical doctors in Chinese culture long before Western cultures.

   _____

   _____

8. True or False? The "father of preventive medicine" was Joseph Lister.

   _____

   _____

9. True or False? Edward Jenner developed the smallpox vaccine in the late 1800s.

   _____

   _____

SELF-ASSESSMENT

1. Make a list of the various ethnic, religious, and cultural groups you and your family members participate in or are descended from.

   _____

   _____

   _____

   _____

2. Interview family members to determine how their ethnic, religious, or cultural beliefs make an impact on the kind of medical care and treatment they expect to receive and how attitudes may have changed or evolved from generation to generation. Write a brief summary of your family's beliefs.

   _____

   _____

   _____

   _____

3. Write down any folk or home remedies used by your parents or grandparents that may or may not still be used by your family today. Why might these remedies have been more widely relied on by previous generations? Is there a scientific basis for each remedy?

   _____

   _____

   _____

   _____

4. An experimental treatment may be the only alternative available for your patient. How would this particular situation affect you, the medical assistant, if it is against your cultural or religious beliefs?

   _____

   _____

   _____

   _____

C H A P T E R **4**

Therapeutic Communication Skills

CHAPTER PRE-TEST

Perform this test without looking at your book. If an answer is "false," rewrite the sentence to make it true.

1. True or False? Gestures and expressions have nothing to do with what a person is thinking or feeling.

   _____

   _____

2. True or False? You can make sick patients "feel better" just by the way you communicate with them.

   _____

   _____

3. True or False? Everyone enjoys a hug.

   _____

   _____

4. True or False? Patients should not be encouraged to verbalize their feelings and concerns.

   _____

   _____

5. True or False? Therapeutic communication can take place without considering the cultural and religious background of the patient.

   _____

   _____

6. True or False? Personal space is the distance at which we feel comfortable with others while communicating.

   _____

   _____

7. True or False? It is not necessary to accept the uniqueness in each person.

_____

_____

8. True or False? It is important for the patient to know that the provider will take the time to listen, answer any questions, and talk with the patient openly.

_____

_____

VOCABULARY BUILDER

Misspelled Words

Find the words below that are misspelled; circle them, and correctly spell them in the spaces provided. Then, insert the correct vocabulary terms from the list that best fits the descriptions below.

active listening	defense mechanisms	perseption
biases	denial	prejidices
body language	encode	rationalization
closed questions	hierarcky of needs	regression
cluster	indirect statements	repression
compinsation	interview technikes	roadblocks
congruancy	kinesics	therapuetic communication
cultural brokering	masking	time focus
decode	open-ended questions	

_____   _____   _____

_____   _____

_____   _____

_____

1. Allows patients to feel comfortable, even when receiving difficult or unpleasant information, achieved through use of specific and well-defined professional communication skills

2. The person seems to experience temporary amnesia; forgetting or wiping things out of the conscious memory

3. Knowing how to encourage the best communication between the health care provider and the patient

4. Human needs grouped into five levels, each level being satisfied first before moving on to the next

5. Types of questions that require only a yes or no answer

6. Verbal or nonverbal messages that prevent patients from expressing themselves

7. The study of nonverbal communication, which includes unconscious body movements, gestures, and facial expressions

_____ 8. Statements that turn a question into a topic of interest that allows the patient to speak without feeling directly questioned

_____ 9. Being aware of what the patient is not saying or the ability to pick up on hints by the patient's body language regarding the real message

_____ 10. Personal preferences slanting toward a particular belief

_____ 11. An opinion or judgment that is formed before all the facts are known

_____ 12. Nonverbal communication that conveys expression or feelings

_____ 13. Types of questions that require more than a yes or no answer, the patient being required to verbalize more information

_____ 14. An attempt to conceal or repress one's true feelings or real message

_____ 15. Nonverbal messages grouped together to form a statement or conclusion

_____ 16. When a person's nonverbal message agrees with that person's verbal message

_____ 17. Interpreting the meaning of the message to understand it

_____ 18. Creation of a carefully crafted message by a sender to match the receiver's ability to receive and interpret it properly

_____ 19. Conscious awareness of one's own feelings and the feelings of others

_____ 20. Substituting a strength for a weakness

_____ 21. The mind's way of making unacceptable behavior or events acceptable by devising a rational reason for it

_____ 22. Refusal to accept painful information that is apparent to others

_____ 23. Attempt to withdraw from an unpleasant circumstance by retreating to a more secure state of life

_____ 24. Act of bridging, linking, or mediating between groups or persons through the process of reducing conflict or producing change

_____ 25. Statements eliciting a response from the patient without the patient's feeling questioned

_____ 26. Unconscious behavior used to protect the ego from guilt, anxiety, or loss of esteem

Crossword Puzzle

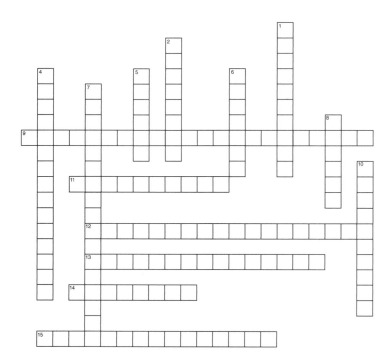

Across

9. Gestures and expressions together with body poses (two words)
11. Moving back to a former stage to escape conflict
12. This "cycle" involves sending and receiving messages, verbal and nonverbal (two words)
13. The art of really hearing another person's message and sometimes verifying with that person what you are hearing
14. The study of body movements
15. Questions that can be answered with a simple yes or no response

Down

1. Opinions or judgments formed before all the facts are known
2. Giving the speaker information about what you are hearing
3. The act of justification, usually illogically, that people use to keep from facing the truth
4. The rejection of or refusal to acknowledge information
5. The position of the body and parts of the body
6. Behavior that protects people from feelings of guilt, anxiety, and shame
7. A slant toward a particular belief
8. Sometimes referred to as temporary amnesia

LEARNING REVIEW

Short Answer

1. List the three listening goals of the health care professional.

_____

_____

_____

2. The four modes of communication most pertinent in our everyday exchange are:

_____

_____

3. Circle the five correct responses. The five Cs of communication are:

clear	coherent	concise
constant	complete	curious
credible	courteous	comment
curt	cooperative	cohesive

4. Understanding Maslow's hierarchy will help medical assistants assess patients' needs and facilitate therapeutic communication. For each level, list a minimum of three needs that meet it.

_____

_____

_____

_____

5. Identify eight significant roadblocks to communication.

_____

_____

_____

6. In order for any type of communication to take place, the patient must trust the health care provider. List the necessary steps in building the patient's trust.

_____

_____

_____

_____

_____

7. How does therapeutic communication differ from normal communication?

_____

_____

8. List and explain the four basic elements included in the communication cycle.

_____

_____

_____

_____

_____

_____

9. Edith Leonard arrives at the clinic for a routine six-month follow-up examination. At her last visit, she had been referred to an ophthalmologist for removal of a cataract in her right eye. Compose (1) a closed question, (2) an open-ended question, and (3) an indirect statement regarding Ms. Leonard's condition.

Closed question:

_____

_____

Open-ended question:

_____

_____

Indirect statement:

_____

_____

10. Time focus relates to whether the patient's attitude toward life is future, present, or past. Fill in the blanks below by explaining what each of these categories mean and list cultures or religions that are oriented to each.

Time focus	Meaning	Cultural or religious groups
Future time focus	_____	_____
	_____	_____
	_____	_____
	_____	_____
Present time focus	_____	_____
	_____	_____
	_____	_____
	_____	_____
Past time focus	_____	_____
	_____	_____
	_____	_____

Matching I

Identify each of the following as high-context communication (H) or low-context communication (L).

____   1. African-American, Western culture

____   2. Relies on highly detailed language to communicate ideas

____   3. Asian culture

____   4. Native American

____   5. Relies on relevant phraseology to communicate ideas

____   6. Caucasian, Western culture

____   7. Hispanic and Latino cultures

____   8. Islam

____   9. Relies on body language to communicate ideas

Matching II

Biases and prejudices common in today's society have the potential to create hostility. Match each difficult situation below to the corresponding bias or prejudice that motivates it. Put a letter in the space provided.

    A. A preference for Western-style medicine

    B. The tendency to choose female rather than male providers

    C. Prejudice related to a person's sexual preference

    D. Discrimination based on race or religion

    E. Hostile attitudes toward persons with a value system opposite to your own

    F. A belief that persons who cannot afford health care should receive less care than those who can pay for full services

____   1. Mr. Gordon refuses to accept a referral to an acupuncturist to help alleviate the chronic pain of advancing prostate cancer.

____   2. Medical assistant Bruce Goldman mistakenly assumes that patient Bill Schwartz has AIDS when he arrives at the clinic with a gentleman friend, seeking attention for a recurring black mole on his calf.

____   3. Rhoda and Lee Au fear they will not receive adequate medical care because they use Chinese as their first language and speak only broken English.

____   4. Corey Boyer resists his gym teacher's efforts to get him to the clinic to check out a recurring rash on his arm because his family has no health insurance.

____   5. Mary O'Keefe is relieved to find that the practice's OB/GYN is a female physician, Dr. Elizabeth King.

____   6. Edith Leonard, a widow in her 70s, counsels medical assistant Liz Corbin that she should settle down and get married instead of pursuing a dream to attend medical school and become a pediatrician.

CERTIFICATION REVIEW

These questions are designed to mimic the certification examination. Select the best response.

1. Which of the following is not part of communication?

  a. Speech

  b. Facial expression

  c. Gestures

  d. Attitude

  e. Body positioning

2. Which is the most basic need in Maslow's hierarchy?

  a. Food

  b. Safety

  c. Status and self-esteem

  d. Need for knowledge

  e. Self-actualization

3. Your patient refuses to accept a diagnosis, claiming the doctor "must be mistaken." Assuming the doctor is correct, which self-defense mechanism is the patient using?

   a. Repression

   b. Denial

   c. Projection

   d. Compensation

   e. Rationalization

4. Congruency in communication can be described as when:

   a. the verbal message matches the body language

   b. the verbal message does not match the gestures

   c. the verbal message can be interpreted in two or more different ways

   d. two different messages are interpreted as the same

5. The conscious awareness of one's own feelings and the feelings of others is:

   a. congruency

   b. perception

   c. bias

   d. masking

6. The founder of humanistic psychology is:

   a. Jacobi

   b. Freud

   c. Erikson

   d. Maslow

7. The grouping of nonverbal messages into statements or conclusions is known as:

   a. assimilating

   b. feedback

   c. clustering

   d. introjection

8. The goal of therapeutic communication at the point of care is:

   a. to collect a blood specimen

   b. to determine the reason for the visit

   c. to explain the treatment plan for the patient

   d. all of the above

LEARNING APPLICATION

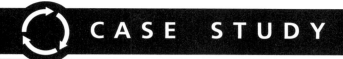

Wayne Elder arrives at the clinic for an examination to check on a recurrent ear infection that has been treated with antibiotics. Wayne, who is slightly retarded and lives in a group home, is still reporting dizziness and pain in his right ear. He has come to the clinic by himself, taking a bus from his job as a part-time dishwasher. Wayne's boss asked him to return to the clinic because Wayne could not concentrate at work.

Wanda Slawson, who is the medical assistant at the clinic, discovers from Wayne that he has not been taking his medication properly; he stopped taking his pills once his ear began to feel better. She must politely ask Wayne to repeat himself several times before she can clearly understand his slurred speech, and she has difficulty holding his attention or maintaining eye contact.

Wanda conveys Wayne's situation to Dr. Ray Reynolds, who examines Wayne and gives him a new prescription for antibiotics, gently explaining the need to finish the entire prescription to get well. After Dr. Reynolds leaves the examination room, however, it is clear to Wanda that Wayne is still confused about why he must take the medication even after he begins to feel better. Wanda carefully explains to Wayne that the infection will continue to heal even though he no longer feels sick. To be sure he understands, Wanda asks Wayne to repeat to her what he must do and why; she then asks Dr. Reynolds to step in briefly to remind Wayne once more to complete the prescription.

CASE STUDY REVIEW QUESTIONS

1. How does the unequal relationship that exists between patients and health care professionals have an impact on the therapeutic communication between provider, medical assistant, and patient?

2. How must medical assistant Wanda Slawson tailor her verbal and nonverbal messages to meet the abilities of her receivers: the provider and the patient?

continues

3. How does Wanda use active listening? Which interview techniques are the most effective in facilitating therapeutic communication? Does nonverbal communication play a role?

    _____

    _____

    _____

    _____

    _____

    _____

    _____

    _____

    _____

    _____

4. Using Maslow's hierarchy of needs, discuss how the health care team meets Wayne's special needs resulting from his disability.

    _____

    _____

    _____

    _____

    _____

    _____

    _____

    _____

5. Do you think the medical assistant acted appropriately? What else could she have done? What should she not do in this situation?

    _____

    _____

    _____

    _____

    _____

Role-Play Exercises

Active listening is an important element of therapeutic communication. To practice active listening skills, role-play as a patient and a medical assistant. Have the "patient" say each of the phrases below. The "medical assistant" should then rephrase each of the messages listed for verification from the sender and also include a therapeutic response. When you are finished role-playing, write what you have said in response to each statement below.

1. "I don't know what to do. My father takes so many pills he can't remember which is the right one, so he ends up refusing to take any of them."

_____

_____

_____

_____

_____

2. "I can't give you my insurance card because I lost it and I can't remember the name of the company, either. You've always taken care of this before."

_____

_____

_____

3. "I can't help being worried. The doctor just suggested a referral for treatment at that hospital where somebody had their wrong foot operated on. What do you think?"

_____

_____

_____

_____

4. "I feel dizzy just thinking about having my blood taken. Do you really need to do it?"

_____

_____

_____

CHAPTER POST-TEST

Perform this test without looking at your book. If an answer is "false," rewrite the sentence to make it true.

1. True or False? Gestures and expressions can always tell you what a person is thinking or feeling.

_____

_____

2. True or False? You can make a sick patient "feel worse" just by the way you communicate with her.

_____

_____

3. True or False? Hugs are universally acceptable as a means of communicating.

_____

_____

4. True or False? Patients should not be allowed to say how they feel or what they are concerned about.

_____

_____

5. True or False? In therapeutic communication, it is not necessary to take into consideration the cultural and religious background of the patient.

_____

_____

6. True or False? The distance at which we feel comfortable while communicating with others is called personal space.

_____

_____

7. True or False? The health care provider should not accept the uniqueness of the patient.

_____

_____

8. True or False? Patients must realize that providers are taking the time to listen to them, answer any of their questions, and speak with them openly.

_____

_____

SELF-ASSESSMENT

Think about your own facial expressions and body language. Are you always portraying the message you want to send? List two situations in which you have been misinterpreted through your nonverbal communication, or situations in which you have misinterpreted someone else's message. Then think of what would have been a verbal message to help make the situation more accurate. That is, explain what you could have said to the person to determine if he or she was really hearing the message you meant to send.

_____

_____

_____

_____

_____

_____

CHAPTER **5**

Coping Skills for the Medical Assistant

CHAPTER PRE-TEST

Perform this test without looking at your book. If an answer is "false," rewrite the sentence to make it true.

1. True or False? Stress is always something bad.

_____

_____

2. True or False? Stress is something we cannot prevent.

_____

_____

3. True or False? If you have a lot of responsibility in your job, you cannot avoid burnout.

_____

_____

4. True or False? Setting goals helps relieve stress.

_____

_____

5. True or False? Goal-oriented employees are more effective than those with no goals or future objectives.

_____

_____

6. True or False? Revitalization outside the workplace is not necessary when preventing burnout.

_____

_____

7. True or False? Worry causes stress but does nothing to resolve the problem that is causing the worry.

_____

_____

VOCABULARY BUILDER

Misspelled Words

Find the words below that are misspelled; circle them, and correctly spell them in the spaces provided. Then insert the vocabulary terms from the list next to their definitions below.

burnout   long-range goal   short-range goal
goal   outer-directed people   stress
inter-directed peepel   self-actualzation   stressers

_____   _____   _____

_____   1. Achievements that may take several years to accomplish

_____   2. Fatigue and exhaustion which results from stress and frustration

_____   3. The body's response to change, which may be manifested in a variety of
                         ways, such as increased blood pressure, heart rate, or headache

_____   4. People who decide what to do based on events, environmental factors, or
                         other people

_____   5. Demands to change that cause stress

_____   6. People who decide for themselves what they want to do

_____   7. Achievement toward which effort has been directed

_____   8. Interim goal that helps to achieve a larger goal over a longer period of time

_____   9. Developing your full potential and experiencing fulfillment

Word Search

Find the words in the grid below. They may go in any direction.

```
T  A  K  E  C  A  R  E  O  F  Y  O  U  R  N  S  E  L  E  F
S  R  O  S  S  E  R  T  S  X  K  L  E  G  O  J  D  M  L  Y
L  L  J  C  K  L  K  K  C  Y  F  L  G  M  I  E  X  R  P  T
T  R  T  F  O  L  F  J  R  G  O  P  W  J  T  X  D  R  O  B
K  H  T  P  H  P  S  G  M  R  T  X  E  Z  A  H  R  S  E  H
L  W  G  R  R  T  I  X  X  Y  N  M  J  M  T  A  F  H  P  H
T  T  F  I  R  I  F  N  T  R  I  G  L  J  P  U  H  O  D  S
H  G  C  E  L  C  O  U  G  T  F  M  L  T  A  S  L  R  E  L
R  R  S  I  R  F  O  R  G  S  F  F  Z  X  D  T  B  T  T  A
M  S  R  R  L  N  R  N  I  R  K  J  K  D  A  I  M  R  C  O
N  C  B  M  R  F  I  O  U  T  L  I  Q  R  T  O  K  A  E  G
N  G  T  U  X  G  N  S  T  Q  I  X  L  L  Y  N  P  N  R  E
Y  Q  B  V  A  C  T  O  R  H  R  Z  H  L  K  Q  Z  G  I  G
T  W  J  N  D  R  Z  C  C  P  G  L  I  Z  S  M  Z  E  D  N
C  R  A  J  A  H  F  F  Z  E  R  I  Z  N  T  H  K  G  R  A
W  M  T  T  J  G  D  V  T  V  L  Q  F  T  G  B  Y  O  E  R
H  Y  I  C  O  N  T  R  O  L  T  O  T  H  N  M  R  A  N  G
Z  O  R  R  S  L  A  O  G  Q  N  T  R  C  M  P  T  L  N  N
N  Z  R  T  J  Z  K  H  N  L  C  V  K  Y  N  M  V  S  I  O
O  U  T  E  R  D  I  R  E  C  T  E  D  P  E  O  P  L  E  L
```

adaptation	frustration	prioritizing
burnout	goals	role
control	inner-directed people	role conflict
coping skills	long-range goals	short-range goals
exhaustion	managing time	stress
fight or flight	outer-directed people	stressors

LEARNING REVIEW

Short Answer

1. Han Selye's general adaptation syndrome (GAS) theory proposes that adaptation to stress occurs in four stages. Identify each stage in the order in which it is manifested and describe the physiologic changes that occur during each stage.

_____

_____

_____

_____

_____

_____

_____

_____

_____

_____

2. Identify six changes in your approach to your work environment and lifestyle that will help you to avoid burnout.

_____

_____

_____

_____

_____

_____

3. List and define the five considerations important in determining a goal.

_____

_____

_____

_____

_____

4. Stressors are divided into three categories. List and describe them.

_____

_____

_____

_____

Matching

Burnout is stress-related energy depletion that takes place in the working world. Burnout occurs gradually over a period of continued stress. Place a P *next to those items that promote burnout and an* R *next to those that reduce the risk for burnout.*

____   1. Keep work separate from your home life.

____   2. Have regular physical examinations.

____   3. Work harder than anyone else in the office.

____   4. Feel a greater need than others to do a job well for its own sake.

____   5. Prioritize tasks and perform the most difficult ones first.

____   6. Prefer to tackle projects yourself rather than consult a supervisor.

____   7. Never stop until you achieve your goals, regardless of the personal cost to yourself or loved ones.

____   8. Postpone vacation time.

____   9. Give up unrealistic goals and expectations.

____   10. Maintain a positive self-image and your self-esteem.

____   11. Develop interests outside your profession.

____   12. Procrastinate.

____ 13. Wear loose-fitting, comfortable clothes and shoes.

____ 14. Stretch or change positions. Walk around and deliver charts or laboratory specimens.

____ 15. Know your limits and be aware of your body's needs.

Labeling

Hans Selye's General Adaptation Syndrome (GAS) theory proposes that four stages are involved in adapting to stress. Identify the four stages on the figure, and then explain each stage in the space below.

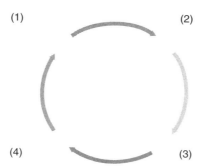

1. _____

2. _____

3. _____

4. _____

CERTIFICATION REVIEW

These questions are designed to mimic the certification examination. Select the best response.

1. The body's response to mental or physical change is called:

   a. stress

   b. adaptation

   c. denial

   d. burnout

2. Which of the following is not part of Hans Selye's general adaptation syndrome?

   a. Exhaustion

   b. Alarm

   c. Fear

   d. Fight or flight

   e. Return to normal

3. The four parts of the process leading to burnout are the honeymoon stage, the reality stage, the dissatisfaction stage, and the:

   a. sad stage

   b. angry stage

   c. retaliation stage

   d. giving up stage

4. In order for the body to survive, the sympathetic nervous system prepares the body for:

   a. fight or flight

   b. sleep

   c. developing a good appetite

   d. exercises

5. Time segments for short-range goals may be:

   a. monthly

   b. quarterly

   c. yearly

   d. all of the above

6. The result of long duration stress could be:

   a. making quick judgments

   b. job related

   c. immune system disorders

   d. an adrenaline rush

7. Stressors can be divided into which category(ies)?

   a. Frustration

   b. Conflicts

   c. Pressure

   d. All of the above

8. Needlessly worrying is an example of which type of stress?

   a. Short-term stress

   b. Episodic stress

   c. Long-term stress

   d. Intermediate stress

9. A common cause of stress in an organization would be:

   a. too much time spent on the telephone

   b. lack of motivation

   c. poor time management skills

   d. no smoke breaks

10. Discipline, perseverance, determination, and hard work are necessary in accomplishing:

    a. short-range goals

    b. long-range goals

    c. self-actualization

    d. prevention of burnout

11. The "wear and tear" our bodies experience as we continually adjust to a changing environment is called:

    a. adaptation

    b. stress

    c. prioritizing

    d. conditioning

12. The fight-or-flight response includes all but which one of the following reactions?

    a. Respirations and heart rate increase.

    b. Digestion is activated.

    c. Hormones are released into the bloodstream.

    d. Blood supply is increased to the muscles.

13. One of the characteristics associated with burnout is that the employee does not know what is expected and how to accomplish it. This is often called:

    a. role conflict

    b. role overload

    c. role ambiguity

    d. role reversal

14. When individuals with a high need to achieve do not reach their goals, they are apt to feel:

    a. angry and frustrated

    b. tired and lonely

    c. distrustful and leery

    d. motivated and enthusiastic

15. The best way to treat burnout is to:

    a. cover it up

    b. get a prescription to help you cope

    c. prevent it

    d. encourage it

LEARNING APPLICATION

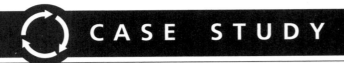

Dr. Angie Esposito is a provider at Inner City Health Care. It was her dream, even as a child, to become a physician and work in an environment where she could help people and benefit the community as well. Proud of her accomplishments, she is the first woman in her family to attend college, and she got herself through medical school with scholarships and student loans. Dr. Esposito works hard, often pulling double shifts. Liz Corbin, CMA (AAMA), has a similar dream and is working to save money to attend medical school to become a pediatrician. Dr. Esposito does her best to encourage Liz's ambitions and has taken Liz under her wing.

Late one night, Liz assists Dr. Esposito in treating three difficult emergency patients in a row. "That's it," Dr. Esposito says. "We're taking a fifteen-minute break. Ask Dr. Woo if he can cover for a short time." When Liz catches up with Dr. Esposito in the employee lounge, she finds her frustrated and in tears. "These double shifts," she says. "I'm so tired. And the patients just keep coming. I want to help them all," she sighs, and her voice trails off, "I just can't help them all. . . ."

CASE STUDY REVIEW QUESTIONS

1. Dr. Angie Esposito is experiencing burnout. What personality traits are promoting her burnout? Identify the stressors in Angie's life.

_____

_____

_____

_____

_____

_____

_____

2. Liz Corbin sees her mentor breaking down under stress. Should Liz reevaluate her own long-range goals?

_____

_____

_____

_____

_____

_____

continues

3. Discuss the importance of keeping goals in perspective.

_____

_____

_____

_____

_____

_____

4. What would be Liz's best therapeutic response to Dr. Esposito?

_____

_____

_____

_____

_____

CHAPTER POST-TEST

Perform this test without looking at your book. If an answer is "false," rewrite the sentence to make it true.

1. True or False? Stress is never a good thing.

_____

_____

2. True or False? Stress is something we can always prevent.

_____

_____

3. True or False? Even if you have a lot of responsibility at work, you can still avoid burnout.

_____

_____

4. True or False? Setting goals eliminates stress.

_____

_____

5. True or False? Those employees who are goal oriented are more effective than those employees who do not have a goal or future objective.

_____

_____

6. True or False? Revitalization outside the workplace is not a contributing factor to burnout.

_____

_____

7. True or False? Worry contributes to stress and does not resolve the problem that is the cause of the worry.

_____

_____

SELF-ASSESSMENT

Determining how well you now handle stress will help you to identify personal strengths and weaknesses and point you toward the skills you will need to develop to be successful on the job as a medical assistant. Complete the following stress self-test. For each question, circle the response that best describes you.

1. I exercise:
    a. three times a week
    b. less than three times a week
    c. only if I am forced to

2. When something stressful happens in my life, I:
    a. eat too much
    b. make sure I eat regular meals
    c. stop eating for days

3. If I am struggling with a problem or project, I am most likely to:
    a. consult someone who may be able to help
    b. become determined to solve the problem or finish the project on my own
    c. abandon the project or just hope the problem goes away

4. When I encounter difficult personalities, I:
    a. leave the scene and avoid the person in the future
    b. lose my temper and get into arguments
    c. practice the art of the diplomatic response

5. When offered a new challenge or responsibility that requires obtaining new skills or training, I:
    a. get tension headaches
    b. respond with enthusiasm and an open mind
    c. express concern about taking on a new duty

6. In emergency situations, I:
    a. react calmly and efficiently
    b. feel paralyzed
    c. wait for someone else to take charge

7. I feel confident and competent in group situations:
    a. only when I know everyone present
    b. most of the time
    c. hardly ever; conversations with others make me uncomfortable

8. I think meditating or taking time to be quiet and calm during a busy day is:

   a. a terrific waste of time; I always have to be doing something

   b. good for other people; I've tried it more than once, but I can't seem to get into meditation

   c. a great way to relax and refocus my mind

9. The key to handling stressful situations lies in:

   a. staying out of stressful situations

   b. examining my view of the situation from a new perspective

   c. insisting that everyone agree with my point of view

10. To accomplish my personal goals, I:

    a. am willing to get up an hour earlier each day

    b. will give up sleep altogether

    c. find myself losing sleep because I am worrying about how I am going to get everything done

11. I usually complete projects:

    a. on time

    b. at the last minute

    c. late—but only by a day

12. As I prepare for a day's activities, I:

    a. prioritize and use time management skills to budget time carefully

    b. do not prepare; I like to be spontaneous

    c. find myself overwhelmed and unable to complete anything

13. When I focus on setting a long-range goal, I:

    a. think through the short-range goals necessary to achieve it

    b. become impatient

    c. talk constantly about the goal without making plans to achieve it

14. I volunteer to take on:

    a. more tasks than any one person can easily accomplish—then amaze everyone by pulling them off

    b. only what I know I can reasonably accomplish

    c. only what is required to get the job done

15. After a stressful day, the best way to unwind is to:

    a. talk all night with family or friends about what happened

    b. rent a funny movie

    c. work late to prepare for tomorrow

16. People think of me as:

    a. a person who is unpredictable. No one knows what I will do next.

    b. someone fixed in life roles

    c. someone who is confident about who I am but who also is willing to grow and change as worthy opportunities arise

Scoring: In the "My Score" column, record the number of points earned for each of your answers. The higher your score, the less you are prone to stress. The highest possible score is 160 points. If your score is low, consider the areas you need to focus on to reduce stress in your life.

MY SCORE

1. a. 10 points b. 5 points c. 0 points
   Regular exercise reduces stress.   _____

2. a. 0 points b. 10 points c. 0 points
   Eating regular meals reduces stress.   _____

3. a. 10 points b. 5 points c. 0 points
   Problems rarely just go away; ask for help before struggling on your own.   _____

4. a. 5 points b. 0 points c. 10 points
   You will not always be able to avoid a difficult person, and argument leads to
   stress. Tact and grace are needed.   _____

5. a. 0 points b. 10 points c. 5 points
   Worrying to the point of causing physical symptoms is not productive. Closed-
   mindedness could keep you from enjoying something new and cause stressful
   reactions.   _____

6. a. 10 points b. 0 points c. 5 points
   Feelings of helplessness increase stress.   _____

7. a. 5 points b. 10 points c. 0 points
   The ability to interact comfortably with others in group situations reduces stress.   _____

8. a. 0 points b. 5 points c. 10 points
   The more you can separate your sense of well-being from daily events by taking
   time to relax and refocus, the less stress you will experience.   _____

9. a. 0 points b. 10 points c. 0 points
   Stressful situations cannot always be avoided; keeping a flexible instead of a rigid
   viewpoint will reduce stress.   _____

10. a. 10 points b. 0 points c. 0 points
    Sleep is important in reducing stress. However, making time by getting up earlier
    is a good time management technique.   _____

11. a. 10 points b. 5 points c. 0 points
    Lateness causes stress for everyone.   _____

12. a. 10 points b. 0 points c. 0 points
    Unexpected things can always happen, but prioritizing and budgeting time can
    help keep a handle on the day's events and reduce stress.   _____

13. a. 10 points b. 5 points c. 0 points
    Achieving long-range goals takes perseverance and determination. Being realistic
    about goals reduces stress.   _____

14. a. 0 points b. 10 points c. 5 points
    Taking on too much responsibility leads to stress.   _____

15. a. 0 points b. 10 points c. 0 points
    Humor is an effective stress reducer—so is separating work from your home life.   _____

16. a. 0 points b. 0 points c. 10 points
    Being grounded but open to new experiences reduces stress.   _____

TOTAL: _____

Areas I need to focus on to reduce stress in my life:

C H A P T E R **6**

The Therapeutic Approach to the Patient with a Life-Threatening Illness

CHAPTER PRE-TEST

Perform this test without looking at your book. If an answer is "false," rewrite the sentence to make it true.

1. True or False? Patients from different cultures will view death and life-threatening illnesses in different ways.

   _____

   _____

2. True or False? The strongest influences in managing life-threatening illnesses in the life of the patient comes from the medical team.

   _____

   _____

3. True or False? Health care professionals are responsible for making sure that patients have all their legal documents in order when diagnosed with a life-threatening illness.

   _____

   _____

4. True or False? Alternative methods of treatment should be discussed with the patient, as well as no treatment at all.

   _____

   _____

5. True or False? When facing a life-threatening illness, setting goals is no longer important.

   _____

   _____

6. True or False? According to Dr. Kübler-Ross, patients go through each of the five states of grief.

_____

_____

VOCABULARY BUILDER

Misspelled Words

Find the words below that are misspelled; circle them, and correctly spell them in the space provided. Then insert the correct vocabulary terms from the list that best fit the descriptions below.

durible power of attorney for health care   living will

health care directive   sychomotor retardation

_____   _____

1. _____ allows the surrogate to make decisions related to health care when the patient is no longer able to do so.

2. A _____ allows patients to make decisions (before becoming incapacitated) of whether life-prolonging medical or surgical procedures are to continue or be withheld.

3. _____ is the slowing of mental responses, decreased alertness, and apathy.

4. A _____ is a legal document that allows a person to make choices related to treatment in a life-threatening illness.

Crossword Puzzle

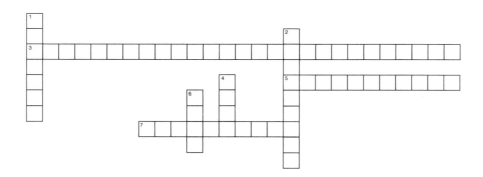

Across
3. This 1990 Act gave all patients in institutions that were Medicare or Medicaid funded certain rights.
5. Aiding health, healthful
7. This emotion is common in patients dealing with life-threatening illnesses.

Down
1. Recognition of another person's feelings by entering into those feelings
2. This type of support is vital when dealing with a life-threatening illness.
4. Late stages of HIV infection (abbreviation)
6. Abbreviation for end-stage renal disease

LEARNING REVIEW

Short Answer

1. List five issues that are appropriate to discuss with a patient facing a life-threatening illness.

   _____

   _____

   _____

2. Discuss the pros and cons of using the words *terminal illness* or *life-threatening illness*. Which term seems more comfortable to you? Defend your rationale.

   _____

   _____

3. The federal government passed the Patient Self-Determination Act in _____, giving all patients receiving care in institutions that receive payments from Medicare and Medicaid written information about their right to accept or refuse medical or surgical treatment.

4. Explain what each of the letters in the acronym TEAR means as it relates to the grieving process.

   T = _____

   E = _____

   A = _____

   R = _____

5. What is the best therapeutic response to the patient with a life-threatening disease?

   _____

   _____

   _____

   _____

True or False

Mark a true statement with a T *and a false statement with an* F. *If an answer is "false," rewrite the sentence to make it true.*

____ 1. It is important for those patients who are suffering from cancer to know that the provider is willing to relieve and treat the symptoms associated with the disease.

   _____

   _____

____ 2. When a person is faced with a life-threatening illness, he or she will go through certain stages of grieving.

   _____

   _____

____ 3. It is not necessary for the health care professional to encourage patients to set goals for themselves.

   _____

   _____

___ 4. It is not necessary to offer nonmedical forms of assistance to patients suffering from a life-threatening illness.

_____

_____

___ 5. All patients go through the five stages of grief.

_____

_____

CERTIFICATION REVIEW

These questions are designed to mimic the certification examination. Select the best response.

1. Your patient's culture influences:

   a. his or her views about illness

   b. his or her views about treatment

   c. his or her views about death

   d. all of the above

2. Your patient has just been diagnosed with a life-threatening illness. She tells you that she would much rather die quickly than to suffer through this disease. She asks you not to say anything about her comment to the doctor. What is your best response?

   a. You have had quite a shock. Dr. King would like to talk to you about those feelings. I'll go get him for you.

   b. You, above anyone else, know what is best for your life.

   c. I know what you mean, I would feel the same way.

   d. Don't worry about that right now. Dr. King will give you medication to help with the pain.

3. The health care directive and power of attorney for health care documents are legal in how many states?

   a. 10

   b. 25

   c. 5

   d. 50

4. The slowing of physical and mental responses, decreased alertness, withdrawal, apathy, and diminished interest in work are referred to as:

   a. passive-aggressive behavior

   b. fight or flight

   c. psychomotor retardation

   d. mood swings

5. The strongest influence in managing the life-threatening illness of a patient is the:

   a. health care team

   b. family and those closest to the patient

   c. social worker

   d. hospice

6. The range of psychological suffering a patient may experience can lead to:

   a. tachycardia

   b. anorexia

   c. agitation

   d. all of the above

7. What patients fear more than anything else when facing a life-threatening illness is:

   a. pain and loss of independence

   b. dementia

   c. financial issues

   d. becoming addicted to some medications

8. In caring for individuals with life-threatening illnesses, it can be helpful to remember:

   a. that family members have the strongest influence on patients

   b. that pain must be considered within a cultural perspective

   c. that choices and decisions regarding treatment belong to the patient

   d. all of the above

9. One of the most common problems that a patient with a life-threatening illness may exhibit is:

   a. displacement

   b. denial

   c. depression

   d. assimilation

10. Referrals to community-based agencies or service groups may include:

    a. health departments

    b. social workers

    c. hospices

    d. all of the above

LEARNING APPLICATION

Role Playing Exercises

With another student, role play the following scenarios as medical assistant and patient. What is the medical assistant's appropriate therapeutic response or action?

1. The patient's husband has just found out that her husband has end-stage renal disease. She tells the medical assistant under no circumstances should her husband be informed about the prognosis.

   _____

   _____

2. The patient has been diagnosed with HIV. The medical assistant knows the patient is estranged from his or her family.

   _____

   _____

CASE STUDY 1

Jaime Carrera, a Hispanic man in his late 20s, is brought to Inner City Health Care, an urgent care center, by coworkers when he injures his head in an accident at a construction site where he is working. His head is bleeding profusely. As Jaime's coworkers watch the health care team implement Standard Precautions for infection control, one of them, his own shirt and hands covered with Jaime's blood, pulls the medical assistant aside and whispers frantically, "What are you doing? Does he have AIDS?"

CASE STUDY REVIEW QUESTIONS

1. What is the best therapeutic response of the medical assistant?

    _____

    _____

    _____

    _____

    _____

    _____

    _____

2. On what criteria do you base this response as the best therapeutic approach?

    _____

    _____

    _____

    _____

    _____

CASE STUDY 2

John Dukane, a longtime and much loved patient of the clinic, has end-stage renal disease. A kidney transplant is not appropriate due to his age, and John will not agree to receiving renal dialysis as treatment. That decision has been made clear in the provider's directive and the durable power of attorney for health care. He is healthy otherwise, and his family members feel he should try the dialysis, in hopes of extending his life by a few weeks or possibly even a few months. Discuss the arguments on both sides of the decision.

_____

_____

_____

_____

CHAPTER POST-TEST

1. True or False? Patients view death and life-threatening illnesses in different ways depending on their culture.

   _____

   _____

2. True or False? The strongest influences in the management of life-threatening illnesses in the life of the patient comes from the health care team.

   _____

   _____

3. True or False? Validating that patients have all their legal documentation in order when diagnosed with life-threatening illness is the responsibility of the health care provider.

   _____

   _____

4. True or False? Alternative methods of treatment, as well as the option of no treatment at all, should be discussed with the patient.

   _____

   _____

5. True or False? When facing a life-threatening illness, setting goals is not important.

   _____

   _____

6. True or False? Patients go through all five of the stages of grief as researched by Dr. Elisabeth Kübler-Ross.

   _____

   _____

SELF-ASSESSMENT

If you were faced with a life-threatening illness, would you choose to sustain your life regardless of the probable outcome? How far would you go with treatments? What four factors would enter into your decision? Have you discussed these issues with your family and physician?

C H A P T E R **9**

Emergency Procedures and First Aid

CHAPTER PRE-TEST

Perform this test without looking at your book. If an answer is "false," rewrite the sentence to make it true.

1. Of the following, which is the most important in an emergency?

   a. Whether the patient has medical insurance

   b. Whether the patient is HIV-positive

   c. Whether the patient is taking any medication

   d. Whether the patient is breathing

2. The abbreviation ABC stands for:

   a. airway, biodynamics, circulation

   b. airway, bleeding, circulation

   c. airway, breathing, circulation

   d. airway, bleeding, cardiac

3. True or False? As a medical assistant, it is important to know how to respond in emergency situations.

   _____

   _____

4. True or False? A first-degree burn is the worst because it has damaged deeper tissues.

   _____

   _____

5. True or False? Whenever a person has a penetrating object embedded in his or her body, it is important that you remove it as soon as possible so you can treat the wound.

   _____

   _____

VOCABULARY BUILDER

Misspelled Words

Find the key vocabulary words below that are misspelled; circle them, and then correctly spell them in the spaces provided.

anaphalaxis   crepidation   occlusion
automated external defibrillator   explicit   sprane
cardioversion   hypothermia   syncopy

_____   _____   _____

_____   _____

Word Search

Find the words in the grid below. They may go in any direction.

```
B E A W A R E E O F Y O U R O W N S A F
E T T R I A G E U Y A S S Y O U C A G Y
R E F O R O T S H C P E R S I N A S R C
N E M E R G P E N R S C Y X X M D T E N
S Y T M L I P R A Z Z E C Q L E Y R E E
Q P H V R Q P I B K K C R H T L S A N G
D C L A R C N W S G Y V O U D M H I S R
N F L I T C O R K Y N G N M Q K O N T E
E D V G N U R V K R N I M X P Q C K I M
G K V N N T V R W I M C H Q X O K T C E
A K L D H M N L S M R D O T W L U D K M
D L S F L M Z S O R J I J P A B T N L Z
N H T T Z C E C P T J A D R E E R D D L
A V G D P R C B R N T T Y Q P R R L K D
B W L R D N D F M Y R S Z T Q K R B D Z
C A R D I A C G W C P R G N I D E E L B
V G E R U T C A R F H I J L N V T Q N N
N O I S S E R P E D L F N K Z J M F M W
F A N A P H Y L A X I S W L N H B N T N
Z D T H Y P O T H E R M I A K T H B K P
```

anaphylaxis   depression   shock
bandage   dressing   spiral
bleeding   emergency   splint
breathing   first aid   sprain
cardiac   fracture   strain
comminuted   greenstick   syncope
compound   hypothermia   wounds
CPR   rescue

LEARNING REVIEW

Matching I

Identify each of the following terms as an emergency condition (EC), an emergency or first aid procedure performed by health care professionals (EP), emergency equipment (EQ), or an emergency service provided to assist in emergency situations (ES).

___   A. First aid

___   B. Screening

___   C. Syncope

___   D. Shock

___   E. Wounds

___   F. Crash cart

___   G. Occlusion

___   H. Universal emergency medical identification symbol and card

___   I. Hypothermia

___   J. Chest Compressions

___   K. CPR

___   L. Sprain

___   M. Emergency medical service (EMS)

___   N. Fracture

___   O. Splints

___   P. Strain

___   Q. Rescue breathing

Matching II

Match each of the terms in Matching I with its definition below.

___   1. A break in a bone. There are several types, but all are classified as open or closed.

___   2. A tray or portable cart that contains medications and supplies needed for emergency and first aid procedures

___   3. An injury to the soft tissue between joints that involves the tearing of muscles or tendons and occurs often in the neck, back, or thigh muscles

___   4. A break in the skin or underlying tissues, categorized as open or closed

___   5. Closure of a passage

___   6. An injury to a joint, often an ankle, knee, or wrist, that involves a tearing of the ligaments. Most are minor and heal quickly; others are more severe, include swelling, and may not heal properly if the patient continues to put stress on the affected joint.

___   7. A local network of police, fire, and medical personnel trained to respond to emergency situations. In most communities, the system is activated by calling 911.

___   8. Identification sometimes carried by individuals to alert to any health problems they might have

___   9. Any device used to immobilize a body part. Often used by EMS personnel

___ 10. An extremely dangerous cold-related condition that can result in death if the individual does not receive care and if the progression of the condition is not reversed. Symptoms include shivering, cold skin, and confusion.

___ 11. Fainting

___ 12. The immediate care provided to persons who are suddenly ill or injured, typically followed by more comprehensive care and treatment

___ 13. A condition in which the circulatory system is not providing enough blood to all parts of the body, causing the body's organs to fail to function properly

___ 14. The combination of rescue breathing and chest compressions performed by a trained individual on a patient experiencing cardiac arrest

___ 15. To assess patients' conditions and prioritize the need for care

___ 16. Performed on individuals in respiratory arrest, this is a mouth-to-mouth (using appropriate protective equipment) or mouth-to-nose procedure that provides oxygen to the patient until emergency personnel arrive.

___ 17. The combination of rescue breathing and this is known as CPR.

Short Answer

1. To identify the nature of the emergency and respond effectively, what five things must the medical assistant do to screen, or assess, the patient's situation?

_____

_____

_____

_____

_____

2. What five infection control measures can health care professionals follow to greatly reduce the risk for transmitting infectious disease when providing emergency care?

_____

_____

_____

_____

_____

3. For each of the patient symptoms or conditions below, identify the type of shock that is most likely.

Patient Symptom/Condition	Type of Shock
Patient suffers heart attack	_____
Patient experiences severe infection after colon surgery	_____
Patient experiences syncope after witnessing a traumatic event	_____
Patient experiences reaction to food allergy	_____
Choking patient has extreme difficulty breathing	_____
Diabetic patient lapses into a coma	_____
Patient has serious head trauma	_____
Accident victim experiences extreme loss of blood	_____

4. A common procedure for treating closed wounds is to RICE them. What do the letters of this acronym stand for?

_____

_____

5. Match each type of open wound (incision, puncture, laceration, avulsion, abrasion) to its defining characteristics.

Characteristics   **Type of Open Wound**

A wound that pierces and penetrates the skin. This wound may appear   _____
insignificant, but actually can go quite deep.

These wounds commonly occur at exposed body parts such as the fingers, _____
toes, and nose. Tissue is torn off and wounds may bleed profusely.

A wound that results from a sharp object such as a scalpel blade.   _____

A painful wound. The epidermal layer of the skin is scraped away.   _____

A wound that results in a jagged tear of body tissues and may contain _____
debris.

6. For each type of wound, describe proper emergency concerns, care, and treatment.

_____

_____

_____

_____

_____

_____

_____

_____

_____

_____

_____

_____

_____

_____

_____

_____

7. Name three sources, other than heat, that can cause burns. For each, describe the proper emergency concerns, care, and treatment.

_____

_____

_____

_____

_____

_____

_____

_____

_____

_____

8. Musculoskeletal injuries, or injuries to muscles, bones, and joints, can be difficult to screen, especially for closed fractures. List five assessment techniques that health care professionals can use to determine the seriousness of musculoskeletal injuries.

_____

_____

_____

_____

9. For each set of symptoms that follows, identify the most likely emergency condition and describe emergency concerns, care, and treatment.

Symptom	Likely Emergency Condition	Emergency Concerns, Care, and Treatment
Off-color, cold skin with a waxy appearance	_____	_____
Hives, itching, lightheadedness	_____	_____

Cold, clammy skin;
profuse sweating;
abdominal cramps;
headache; general
weakness

_____ _____
                  _____
                  _____
                  _____
                  _____
                  _____

Lightheadedness,
weakness, nausea,
unsteadiness

_____ _____
                  _____
                  _____
                  _____
                  _____
                  _____

Moist, pale skin;
drooling; lack of
appetite; diplopia;
full pulse

_____ _____
                  _____
                  _____
                  _____
                  _____
                  _____

Numbness in face,
arm, and leg on one
side of body; slurred
speech; nausea and
vomiting, loss of
vision, severe
headache, mental
confusion, difficulty
breathing and
swallowing

_____ _____
                  _____
                  _____
                  _____
                  _____

Convulsions,
clenched teeth

_____ _____
                  _____
                  _____
                  _____
                  _____

Cold, clammy skin; _____ _____
rapid, weak pulse;
low blood pressure, _____ _____
shallow breathing;
dizziness, faintness, _____
thirst, restlessness, _____
feeling of anxiety;
abdomen may be stiff _____
and hard to the touch _____

10. Identify the method of entry into the body for each of the following poisons:

_____ 1. Carbon monoxide

_____ 2. Insect stingers

_____ 3. Chemical pesticides used in the garden

_____ 4. Spoiled food

_____ 5. Poison oak

_____ 6. Cleaning fluid fumes

CERTIFICATION REVIEW

These questions are designed to mimic the certification examination. Select the best response.

1. Which of the following is not an appropriate treatment for hypothermia?

   a. Give the victim warm liquids to drink.

   b. Remove any wet clothing.

   c. Rub the victim's skin vigorously to increase circulation.

   d. Use warm water to warm the person if possible.

2. In anaphylactic shock, the patient will:

   a. feel a constriction in the throat and chest

   b. have difficulty breathing

   c. have swelling and tingling of the lips and tongue

   d. All of the above

3. While waiting for EMS to arrive, what should be checked?

   a. Degree of responsiveness

   b. Airway, breathing

   c. Heartbeat (rate and rhythm)

   d. All of the above

4. Closed wounds that are painful and swollen require that a cold compress be applied:

   a. until the victim feels tingling

   b. for 10 minutes, then off for 40 minutes

   c. for 20 minutes, then off for 20 minutes

   d. for at least 1 hour, then off for 2 hours

5. To control nosebleeds, the patient should be seated, the patient's head elevated, and nostrils pinched for:

   a. 10 minutes

   b. 20 minutes

   c. 30 minutes

   d. 40 minutes

6. When a patient calls regarding a poisoning or suspicion of poisoning, the advice to give is to:

   a. call the poison control center

   b. give the patient charcoal

   c. tell the patient to drink milk

   d. flush the mouth with water

7. The best treatment for patients who are experiencing a seizure is to:

   a. restrain them

   b. stick a tongue depressor in their mouth

   c. protect from injury and care for them with understanding

   d. stop the seizure

8. Shock that occurs as a result of overwhelming emotional factors such as fear, anger, or grief is called:

   a. neurogenic

   b. psychogenic

   c. anaphylactic

   d. septic

9. The type of burn that may occur resulting in an entrance and exit burn wound area is:

   a. chemical

   b. electrical

   c. solar radiation

   d. explosion

10. In burn depth classifications, third-degree burns are also called:

    a. superficial

    b. full thickness

    c. partial thickness

    d. sunburns

11. The type of fracture often caused by falling on an outstretched hand that involves the distal end of the radius is called:

    a. greenstick

    b. spiral

    c. Colles

    d. implicated

12. Jaw and left shoulder pain; a rapid, weak pulse; excessive perspiration; and cold, clammy skin may be symptomatic of:

   a. seizure

   b. heart attack

   c. stroke

   d. sepsis

LEARNING APPLICATION

Screening Activity

In an urgent care setting, two or more patients may present with emergency symptoms. The order in which emergency patients will receive care depends on the health care professionals' abilities to screen patients' symptoms to determine who needs care most urgently. The following five patients present simultaneously on New Year's Eve at Inner City Health Care, an urgent care center. Office manager Walter Seals, CMA (AAMA), is working the evening shift with Dr. Mark Woo. In what order will Walter and Mark screen the priority of treatment? Number the patients 1 (most urgent) through 5 to correspond to the urgency of their conditions.

Patient	**Urgency**
Patient A presents with a gunshot wound to the leg that is bleeding severely. The patient is conscious but his pupils are dilated and he is unable to answer simple questions put to him by Walter and Dr. Woo. He cradles his right arm and will not let anyone touch it, although there is no immediate evidence of an open wound to the arm.	_____
Patient B, an elderly man, is brought in by his grandson. He describes debilitating chest pains, difficulty breathing, and nausea after eating a large family dinner. The patient's medical record indicates that he has a hiatal hernia, slipped disks, high blood pressure, and mild angina. The man is walking and speaking with moderate distress and is extremely anxious.	_____
Patient C, a young woman, presents with her boyfriend. She appears to have multiple abrasions on her right palm and knee, with damage to the right knee and ankle joints sustained after a fall while on in-line skates. Both joints are swollen and painful.	_____
Patient D, a man in his mid-30s, presents with the cotton tip of a swab stuck in his ear canal. Although the man feels a dull consistent pain in the ear, he says he has no trouble hearing. The outside of the ear appears normal, there is no bleeding evident, and the man appears annoyed but not distressed.	_____
Patient E, a young woman, presents with a group of friends, all college students, with an eye injury sustained by a champagne cork. The cork, which had a metal covering over its tip, hit the patient's eye. The young woman's eye is red and tearing and she is experiencing severe pain in the eye.	_____

CASE STUDY 1

Mary O'Keefe calls Dr. King's office in a panic. Ellen Armstrong, CMA (AAMA), answers the telephone.

Mary: "Oh my God, help me. I need Dr. King."

Ellen: "This is Ellen Armstrong. Who is this calling? What is the situation?"

Mary: "It's my baby, oh God, get Dr. King."

Ellen: "Dr. King is unavailable, but we can help you. Now, tell me your name."

Mary: "It's Mary O'Keefe. Help me, I think my baby is dead."

Ellen: "Are you at home?"

Mary: "Yes."

Ellen: "Good. Tell me what's happened."

Mary: "My son Chris pried the plug off an outlet and he's electrocuted himself!" Mary cries. "He's just lying there. I'm so scared, if I touch him, will I electrocute myself? Oh my God, my baby, my baby. What should I do?"

Ellen, who has been writing down the details on a piece of paper, motions to Joe Guerrero, another CMA (AAMA) in the office, and hands him her notes. Joe immediately accesses the O'Keefe address from the patient database and uses another telephone to call EMS with the nature of the emergency situation and directions to the O'Keefe residence. Meanwhile, Ellen remains on the line with Mary. Dr. King is on rounds at the hospital this morning and will not be in the office for at least another hour.

Ellen: "Mary, we are calling EMS, and they will be there as soon as possible. In the meantime, I'm going to need you to focus and answer my questions, okay?"

CASE STUDY REVIEW QUESTIONS

1. What steps did the medical assistant take to screen the emergency situation?

_____

_____

_____

_____

_____

_____

2. What questions should Ellen ask Mary regarding the emergency situation?

_____

_____

_____

_____

_____

continues

3. What should the medical assistant do after EMS arrives and takes over emergency care? What follow-up procedures are necessary?

_____

_____

_____

_____

_____

_____

_____

_____

_____

_____

_____

CASE STUDY 2

Lenore McDonell, a wheelchair-bound woman in her early 30s, experiences a serious laceration to the right arm sustained from a fall while performing an independent transfer from the examination table to her wheelchair. Joe Guerrero, CMA (AAMA), assists Dr. Winston Lewis in administering emergency care.

CASE STUDY REVIEW QUESTIONS

1. What Standard Precautions must the health care professionals follow before administering emergency treatment?

_____

_____

_____

2. Joe and Dr. Lewis attempt to control Lenore's bleeding by applying a dressing and pressing firmly. When the bleeding does not stop, what two actions should the health care professionals perform?

_____

_____

continues

3. In the unlikely event that bleeding continues, what piece of medical equipment will the health care team use in substitution for a tourniquet? Why is this alternative equipment effective and widely used today?

_____

_____

_____

_____

_____

_____

4. The bleeding stops, and Joe applies a pressure bandage over the dressing. This patient is prone to fractures, and a radiograph will need to be taken. What is the next emergency procedure Dr. Lewis will perform? Why is this procedure necessary, and what equipment will the provider and medical assistant require?

_____

_____

_____

_____

_____

5. Before applying a sling, what do the health care professionals check to be sure that the medical equipment used has not been too tightly applied?

_____

_____

_____

6. What Standard Precautions will the health care team follow after the emergency treatment of the patient is successfully completed?

_____

_____

_____

7. What information will the health care team include in documenting the procedure for the patient's medical record?

_____

_____

_____

_____

_____

Research Activity

Using a medical encyclopedia or reference such as the *Physician's Desk Reference* (PDR), describe the following emergency medications and identify potential uses for each. Remember that only a provider can order medications or treatment.

Lidocaine: _____

_____

Verapamil: _____

_____

Atropine: _____

_____

_____

_____

Insulin: _____

_____

Nitroglycerin: _____

_____

Marcaine: _____

_____

Diphenhydramine: _____

_____

Diazepam: _____

_____

CHAPTER POST-TEST

Perform this test without looking at your book. If an answer is "false," rewrite the sentence to make it true.

1. Of the following, which is the most important in an emergency?

   a. Whether the patient has medical insurance

   b. Whether the patient is HIV-positive

   c. Whether the patient is taking any medication

   d. Whether the patient is breathing

2. ABC stands for:

   a. airway, biodynamics, circulation

   b. airway, bleeding, circulation

   c. airway, breathing, circulation

   d. airway, bleeding, cardiac

3. True or False? As a medical assistant, you should be prepared to respond to small-scale and large-scale emergency situations.

_____

_____

4. True or False? A first-degree burn is the worst because it has damaged deeper tissues.

_____

_____

5. True or False? Whenever a penetrating object has been embedded in a person's body, it is important that you remove it as soon as possible so you can treat the wound.

_____

_____

SELF-ASSESSMENT

1. A. On a scale of 1 to 5, rate your personal comfort in regard to the following emergency situations that medical assistants may find themselves involved with in an ambulatory or urgent care setting.

1 = extremely uncomfortable   4 = comfortable

2 = uncomfortable   5 = very comfortable

3 = somewhat comfortable

_____ Assisting in treatment of patients with injuries clearly sustained by an act of violence or abuse

_____ Administering back blows and thrusts to a conscious infant

_____ Performing rescue breathing on someone who has poor personal hygiene

_____ Bandaging the open wound of an HIV-infected person

_____ Caring for a person experiencing a seizure

_____ Administering care to a patient who faints after venipuncture

_____ Administering care to a patient in extreme pain

_____ Administering care to a patient who is verbally abusive or uncooperative

2. On a scale of 1 to 5, rate your level of agreement with the statements that follow.

    1 = never   4 = most of the time

    2 = occasionally   5 = all of the time

    3 = sometimes

_____ Life-threatening emergencies frighten me.

_____ I respond well under pressure.

_____ I am bothered by the sight of blood.

_____ I lose my temper easily, becoming openly frustrated and angry.

_____ I become frustrated and overwhelmed by feelings of helplessness in emergency situations.

_____ I remain calm and clearheaded in emergency situations.

_____ I forget about myself completely and focus on the emergency victim.

_____ I am concerned about administering care in emergency situations in which danger to myself may exist when giving such care.

_____ I am comfortable speaking to the family or friends of emergency victims.

C H A P T E R **10**

Creating the Facility Environment

CHAPTER PRE-TEST

Perform this test without looking at your book. If an answer is "false," rewrite the sentence to make it true.

1. A reception area should:

    a. be comfortable and inviting

    b. be clean and uncluttered

    c. contain current reading materials for all ages

    d. All of the above

2. True or False? It is considerate, but not required, to provide at least one handicapped patient parking space.

    _____

    _____

3. Keeping the reception area clean is a responsibility of:

    a. the adminstrative medical assistant

    b. the bookkeeper

    c. the laboratory technician

    d. the office manager

    e. All of the above

4. True or False? Cultural differences will also have an impact on the amount of space necessary for the reception area.

    _____

    _____

VOCABULARY BUILDER

Misspelled Words

Find the words below that are misspelled; circle them, and correctly spell them in the spaces provided. Then insert vocabulary terms from the list that best fit into the descriptive sentences below.

accessibility   Americans with Disibilities Act   enviroment
accountibility   characteristic

_____   _____   _____

_____   1. The physical space of the reception area

_____   2. A typical or distinguishing quality

_____   3. Being ultimately responsible

_____   4. Being readily reachable

_____   5. Mandates that facilities and equipment be available to all users

Word Search

Find the words in the grid below. They may go in any direction.

```
L  S  C  I  T  A  M  R  O  F  N  I  O  O  P  E
K  E  A  T  Y  F  A  C  I  L  I  T  Y  L  S  N
O  U  L  R  R  E  C  E  P  G  T  I  A  O  C  V
N  A  R  B  E  A  A  S  N  A  A  Y  P  G  I  I
A  D  E  L  A  Y  S  I  T  C  I  T  E  N  T  R
N  T  W  O  U  T  D  L  C  D  S  V  I  I  S  O
D  E  L  W  A  A  R  E  I  I  T  .  F  T  I  N
T  E  F  I  E  A  S  O  N  K  T  K  V  I  R  M
J  J  S  R  G  S  P  O  F  G  P  B  T  V  E  E
F  N  N  I  I  H  I  I  N  M  T  Y  T  N  T  N
R  N  Z  B  G  T  T  I  H  K  O  M  O  I  C  T
L  D  L  H  P  N  M  I  Z  Z  R  C  Y  A  A  V
K  E  V  E  L  L  H  B  N  Z  N  Q  S  D  R  K
N  T  C  W  A  G  P  L  Q  G  M  Z  M  A  A  L
R  E  L  C  B  G  N  I  M  O  C  L  E  W  H  V
R  K  M  N  R  F  U  R  N  I  T  U  R  E  C  G
```

accessible   design   play
ADA   environment   reading
calming   facility   reception
characteristics   furniture   toys
comfortable   inviting   welcoming
delays   lighting

LEARNING REVIEW

Short Answer

1. What is the purpose of the ADA?

_____

_____

_____

2. When creating the facility environment, why is accessibility a major consideration?

_____

_____

_____

_____

3. Why are some medical clinics experimenting with the use of water, such as aquariums and water walls, and music in their facilities?

_____

_____

_____

_____

4. Name four ways an ambulatory care setting can accommodate the physically challenged.

_____

_____

_____

5. Identify at least four things to be done in the reception area to accommodate children.

_____

_____

_____

6. List at least five safety and evacuation considerations in the medical office.

_____

_____

_____

_____

_____

7. Create a checklist of five activities to perform on opening a medical facility for the day.

_____

_____

_____

8. Create a checklist of five activities to perform on closing a medical facility for the day.

_____

_____

_____

_____

9. Any drugs identified in the Controlled Substance Act list of narcotics and non-narcotics must be *(circle all that apply)*:

   a. logged

   b. in a locked and secured cabinet

   c. checked when leaving the office

   d. counted

10. In each of the following situations, health care professionals should strive to empower the patient with as much control and dignity as possible.

    Case 1. Bill Schwartz is referred to a dermatologist by Dr. Ray Reynolds for examination of a suspicious mole on his calf. The dermatologist tells Bill that a full-body inspection will need to be done to ensure that no other areas of the skin are affected. Bill must appear disrobed in front of the dermatologist and medical assistant, who are both female.

    What strategies can health care professionals use to respect the patient's dignity and lessen the sense of disproportion between health care providers and the patient?

    _____

    _____

    _____

    _____

    _____

    Case 2. Ellen Armstrong, CMA (AAMA), places a Holter monitor on patient Charles Williams. After the Holter monitor is in place, Charles has several questions about the patient activity diary that he would prefer to discuss with Dr. Winston Lewis.

    What strategies can health care professionals use to respect the patient's dignity and lessen the sense of disproportion between health care providers and the patient?

    _____

    _____

    _____

    _____

    _____

    _____

    _____

Physical Office Environment Review

The physical clinic environment can contribute to the patient's sense of confidence and comfort, or it can be viewed by the patient as intimidating or anxiety producing. For each clinic area below, describe why the area could be perceived by patients as a frightening place. What can be done to make each area a more comforting and welcoming environment for patients?

A. Reception area:

_____

_____

_____

_____

_____

B. Corridors:

_____

_____

_____

_____

_____

C. Examination rooms:

_____

_____

_____

_____

_____

_____

_____

Fill in the Blanks

Fill in the blanks in the sentences below, which discuss the future environment for ambulatory care.

1. Patients who are 85 years or older and who are most likely to require medical care for multiple chronic conditions is expected to increase by _____ by 2010.

2. The number of primary care providers willing to take new patients who are 65 years or older must _____.

3. _____ requires providers to have patients sign a release so the family members can be kept informed.

4. The greatest frustration of elderly patients regarding their health care experiences is the _____ _____ given by all health professionals.

5. It is important to provide clear and concise _____ instructions whenever possible in easy-to-read print.

6. The medical environment should enable all patients to _____ from one department to another with ease.

CERTIFICATION REVIEW

These questions are designed to mimic the certification examination. Select the best response.

1. HIPAA has changed the way we organize our entrance and reception areas in the following way:

    a. Patients must be able to see the receptionist at all times.

    b. Patients must have adequate parking.

    c. Patients must not be able to see or hear confidential information about other patients.

    d. The magazines must be current.

2. ADA states that:

    a. Patients must not know the names and diagnoses of other patients.

    b. Handicapped patients must have access to all patient areas with reasonable accommodations.

    c. Visually impaired patients must have adequate lighting and contrast for better viewing.

    d. An interpreter must be present with any non–English-speaking patient.

3. Patient safety within the reception area is accomplished by:

    a. providing chairs that are sturdy and in good repair

    b. containing wires and cords and keeping them out of reach

    c. attaching rugs to the flooring without loose edges

    d. containing toys within a designated play area

    e. All of the above

4. The reception area should accommodate:

    a. at least one hour's patients per provider plus a friend or relative who may accompany each patient

    b. only adult patients

    c. 2.5 seats for each examination room

    d. a. and c.

5. Before entering the exam room, health care professionals should:

    a. turn their cell phones off

    b. knock before entering

    c. wash their hands

    d. put on lab coats

6. According to the ADA, there must be one accessible entrance that should:

    a. have a padlock

    b. state that it is an exit

    c. have a doorbell

    d. be protected from the weather by a canopy or overhanging roof

7. The administrative medical assistant should be able to:

    a. perform telephone screening

    b. remember that the patient's comfort is of primary concern

    c. log data into the computer

    d. All of the above

8. A good way to check a room's readiness is to:

   a. lie on the examining table and look around

   b. place yourself in the room as a patient

   c. ask yourself how you feel about being there and what mood the surroundings create for you

   d. b. and c.

9. When closing the facility for the day, it is most important to:

   a. contact the answering service to notify them that the office is closed and who can be reached in an emergency

   b. clean all rooms

   c. lock the doors

   d. turn off the lights

10. Making facilities and equipment available to all users is called:

    a. maintenance

    b. accessibility

    c. promotion

    d. standardization

11. HIPAA requires that clinic facilities:

    a. have adequate corridors and bathrooms to accommodate wheelchair patients

    b. place an administrative medical assistant in an area seen and heard by all patients

    c. protect the confidentiality of patients checking in at the reception desk

    d. provide space for children in the clinic

12. The primary goal of maintaining a comfortable environment in which patient care is given is to:

    a. feed anxiety

    b. aggravate illness

    c. promote health

    d. stimulate the senses

13. Space planners suggest:

    a. that the reception area accommodate at least two hours' patients per provider

    b. that the reception area accommodate a friend or relative who might accompany each patient

    c. that there be 2.5 seats in the reception area for each examination room

    d. only b. and c.

14. Any drugs kept in the office that are identified as controlled substances must always be kept:

    a. in the refrigerator

    b. in a locked, secure cabinet

    c. in the provider's desk drawer

    d. in the administrative medical assistant's desk drawer

LEARNING APPLICATION

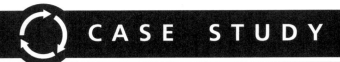

CASE STUDY

Lydia Renzi, a near-deaf woman with some residual hearing, is a patient of Dr. Angie Esposito's at Inner City Health Care. Lydia is fluent in American Sign Language (ASL) and usually wears a hearing aid when she is away from home. Lydia calls to make her appointment at Inner City Health Care using a telecommunications device for the deaf (TDD) and the services of a government-funded relay operator. Although Lydia often chooses not to be accompanied by an interpreter, Inner City Health Care always provides the option to supply the services of a qualified professional sign language interpreter in compliance with the ADA. When Lydia arrives at Inner City Health Care with a high fever and a suspected case of the flu, the staff accommodates Lydia's special needs in several simple ways. Remembering that people who are hearing impaired rely on visual images to receive and to convey messages, Liz Corbin, CMA (AAMA), always faces Lydia directly so that the patient can see her facial expressions and lip movements. Liz holds eye contact with Lydia and does not break it until she is sure that Lydia understands her message and has time to think and respond. Special care is taken to provide Lydia with written instructions for prescriptions and for following through on home care.

CASE STUDY REVIEW QUESTIONS

1. What are the special communication needs of the hearing-impaired patient in the ambulatory care setting?

   _____

   _____

   _____

   _____

   _____

   _____

   _____

   _____

   _____

   _____

2. How can the medical assistant's actions make a direct impact on the quality of care given to hearing-impaired patients?

   _____

   _____

   _____

   _____

   _____

   _____

continues

3. Suppose that Lydia is an elderly woman who is embarrassed and sensitive about her hearing loss and will not admit that she has trouble hearing others. How might the medical assistant accommodate the special needs of this patient?

_____
_____
_____
_____
_____
_____
_____

Role-Play Exercises

The administrative medical assistant is the person who sets the social climate for the interchange between the patient and the health care team. A friendly, reassuring demeanor and an ability to screen situations are essential skills. With another student, role-play as a patient and an administrative medical assistant. Have the "patient" say each of the phrases below. When you are finished role-playing, write what you have said and done in response to each statement below.

1. A patient with intense stomach pain doubles over and then bolts up to the reception desk, saying, "I'm going to throw up."

_____
_____
_____
_____
_____
_____
_____

2. When presented with a bill, the patient exclaims, "I can't pay for all of this now! Every time I come here it seems like the doctor bill goes up a hundred dollars."

_____
_____
_____
_____
_____
_____

3. A patient is looking for the correct exit from the examination area to the waiting area and makes a wrong turn into the administrative medical assistant's area. He asks, "Where do I go?"

_____
_____
_____
_____

4. A patient new to an HMO plan does not realize that a separate referral form is needed for a follow-up visit with the gastroenterologist one week after a colonoscopy test has been performed. She says, "I drove an hour to get to this appointment. No one told me I needed another form."

_____

_____

_____

_____

_____

_____

_____

_____

_____

CHAPTER POST-TEST

Perform this test without looking at your book. If an answer is "false," rewrite the sentence to make it true.

1. A reception area should:

   a. be comfortable, clean, and uncluttered

   b. contain current reading materials for all ages

   c. have adequate lighting for reading

   d. contain accommodations for patients with disabilities

   e. All of the above

2. True or False? It is required to provide one handicapped patient parking space.

   _____

   _____

3. Keeping the reception area clean is a responsibility of:

   a. the administrative medical assistant

   b. the bookkeeper

   c. the laboratory technician

   d. the office manager

   e. all employees

4. True or False? Cultural differences do have an effect regarding the amount of space necessary for the reception area.

   _____

   _____

SELF-ASSESSMENT

1. Visualize your last visit to a medical facility. Was the reception area clean, tidy, welcoming, and comfortable? What would you do to improve it?

   _____

   _____

   _____

2. List at least three things you would add to any reception area to make it even more accommodating. Think of items not mentioned in the textbook.

   _____

   _____

   _____

   _____

   _____

C H A P T E R **1 1**

Computers in the Ambulatory Care Setting

CHAPTER PRE-TEST

Perform this test without looking at your book. If an answer is "false," rewrite the sentence to make it true.

1. The keyboard and the mouse are considered to be:

    a. the most common types of input device

    b. the most common types of output device

    c. portable memory storage devices

    d. read-write devices

2. To ensure that your work in the computer is safe from hackers, you should:

    a. store all work on data storage devices

    b. defragment frequently

    c. use firewalls

    d. backup frequently

3. Circle each of the following tasks that are performed by a computer as part of a total practice management system:

    a. Keeping track of appointments

    b. Writing and forwarding prescriptions to the patient's pharmacy

    c. Creating patient statements

    d. Processing insurance claims

    e. Reading directions on how to download a software program

4. The "brain" of the computer is called the:

   a. motherboard

   b. modem

   c. video card

   d. central processing unit (CPU)

5. To prevent unauthorized use of your clinic computers, you should:

   a. keep the computer in a locked cabinet at all times

   b. keep the computer in a locked cabinet at night

   c. assign every employee a password

   d. have only one person on the computer at a time

VOCABULARY BUILDER

Misspelled Words

Find the words below that are misspelled; circle them, and correctly spell them in the spaces provided. Then insert the correct vocabulary terms from the list that best fit the descriptions below.

electronic medical records	hardware	RAM
erganomics	Internet	total practice management
fishing	modom	system

_____

_____ 1. A device used by a computer to communicate to a remote computer through phone lines

_____ 2. Maximizing the user's safety when setting up a workstation that involves preventing back, neck, and eye strain

_____ 3. Acronym for *random access memory*, a type of computer memory that can be written to and read from

_____ 4. The physical equipment used by the computer system to process data

_____ 5. The practice of attempting to acquire sensitive information (such as passwords or bank account numbers) by masquerading as a trusted source through email communication

_____ 6. Electronic patient records from a single medical practice, hospital, or pharmacy

_____ 7. A worldwide computer network available via modem

_____ 8. A category of software that deals with the day-to-day operations of a medical practice

Crossword Puzzle

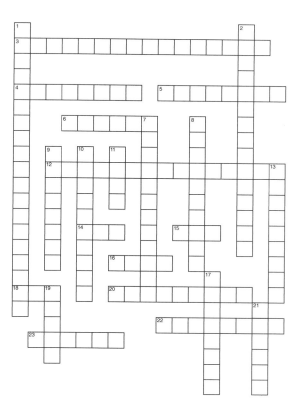

Across

3. Also known as a microcomputer
4. A worldwide computer network available via modem
5. Components of a computer system that you can touch, see, or hear
6. A unit composed of a number of parts that function together to perform a particular task
12. Software that provides instructions to the computer hardware and also runs computer programs
15. Acronym for *read only memory*
16. Amount of memory needed to store one character
18. Stores in-progress data and is the acronym for *random access memory*
20. Nonportable storage device that is read-write with permanent memory
22. Hardware connections that are made using a crossover cable between computers that have an installed network interface controller
23. Storage device for workstations

Down

1. Software that performs a specific data processing function
2. Removes blank spaces left from deleted files
7. Processes data in health care facilities such as patient account processing, insurance claim processing, and statistical analysis of research data
8. A readily transportable data storage device that moves data between computers that are not connected on a network
9. Frequently referred to as a computer program
10. Electronic or optical connection of computers and peripheral equipment for the purpose of sharing information and resources
11. The raw material and collection of characters and numbers entered into a computer
13. A large computer system used for large volumes of repetitive calculations and for governmental provider service programs such as Medicare and Medicaid
17. Allows site access to your computer
19. An input or output device which alters digital data from the computer and transmits it over telephone lines
21. Data storage device capacity

LEARNING REVIEW

Short Answer

1. List the tasks that should be performed by members of the health care team when maintaining the computer.

   _____

   _____

   _____

2. What precautions must be taken to ensure that data are not lost during a power outage?

   _____

   _____

   _____

3. What are the three most common networks encountered in the medical office?

   _____

   _____

4. Name several hardware connections to a network.

   _____

   _____

5. Name several wireless connections to a network.

   _____

   _____

6. Name the two different techniques used by antivirus software to scan files to identify and eliminate computer viruses and malware.

   _____

   _____

   _____

7. List at least six of the defenses that should be used in protecting the health care facility's computer system.

   _____

   _____

   _____

   _____

8. The four fundamental elements of all computer systems are:

   _____

   _____

9. List the HIPAA compliance measures to be taken that will ensure that all PHI data are accurate and not altered, lost, or destroyed.

   _____

   _____

   _____

   _____

10. The identifying characteristics of a secure site are *(circle all that apply)*:

    a. small padlock icon in the Web browser window

    b. site address: https://

    c. an "S" in the upper left corner of the screen

    d. site address: http://

11. What is meant by "electronic medical record" and "electronic health record"? Distinguish between the terms.

    _____

    _____

    _____

    _____

CERTIFICATION REVIEW

These questions are designed to mimic the certification examination. Select the best response.

1. A flash drive is a:

    a. memory device

    b. type of software device

    c. DVD drive

    d. safety warning

2. What step(s) should be followed when selecting software?

    a. Choose a knowledgeable vendor.

    b. Determine what tasks will be computerized.

    c. Software available for each task should be identified and evaluated on a trial basis.

    d. All of the above

3. A personal digital assistant is classified as a:

    a. supercomputer

    b. mainframe computer

    c. minicomputer

    d. microcomputer

4. Computers in the medical office or clinic are used to perform:

    a. routine office tasks

    b. maintenance of electronic medical records and management of the clinic or practice

    c. clinical laboratory applications

    d. a. and b. only

    e. a., b., and c.

5. Defragmenting gets rid of:

   a. fragments of information that you do not need anymore

   b. old information no longer needed

   c. empty spaces on the hard drive

   d. removal of software that you do not use

6. The fastest, most complex, and most expensive computer that is also used in medical research is the:

   a. mainframe

   b. supercomputer

   c. minicomputer

   d. personal digital assistant

7. The smallest but most widely used type of computer in today's heath care facility is the:

   a. microcomputer

   b. supercomputer

   c. mainframe computer

   d. minicomputer

8. Examples of output devices would be:

   a. printers, fax machines, monitors

   b. keyboard, mouse

   c. scanners, electronic tablets

   d. touch screens, digital cameras

9. What step(s) should be taken in the changeover to a computer system?

   a. Schedule during a down period, such as a long holiday or vacation period.

   b. Introduce the new system while continuing to use the old system.

   c. Transfer files and data and when the staff is comfortable with the system and their computer skills, then make the changeover.

   d. All of the above

10. Manuals and documents that define how programs operate are called:

    a. the operating system

    b. system software

    c. computer system documentation

    d. application software

11. Compact disks and digital video versatile disks are two types of

    a. hard drives

    b. optical drives

    c. flash drives

    d. tape drives

12. Data storage device capacity is often referred to as

    a. hardware

    b. the operating system

    c. memory

    d. algorithms

13. Portable memory storage devices from which the storage media can be readily removed and transported are called:

    a. flash drives

    b. ROM

    c. RAM

    d. optical drives

LEARNING APPLICATION

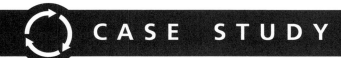

CASE STUDY

Due to an influx of patient volume, the practice of Drs. Lewis and King will have to hire more administrative staff and expand their office space. Three more computers have been installed, with updated software programs. Shirley Brooks, CMA (AAMA), practice manager, is trying to avoid any future safety issues in the workplace.

CASE STUDY REVIEW QUESTION

1. What factors should she take into consideration when setting up each workstation to be "ergonomically correct"?

   _____

   _____

   _____

   _____

   _____

   _____

   _____

   _____

   _____

   _____

   _____

CHAPTER POST-TEST

Perform this test without looking at your book. If an answer is "false," rewrite the sentence to make it true.

1. The most common type of input device is the:

   a. USB port

   b. flash drive

   c. monitor

   d. keyboard

2. To ensure that your computer information is safe from unauthorized viewing within the office:

   a. use firewalls

   b. defragment frequently

   c. use passwords

   d. back up frequently

3. Which of the following is *not* a function of a total practice management system?

   a. Keeping track of appointments

   b. Keeping track of accounts receivable

   c. Keeping track of accounts payable

   d. Processing insurance claims

   e. Reading directions on how to download software

4. Part of the system that carries out instructions defined by the program software or the data input then sends the results to the selected output devices is called the:

   a. motherboard

   b. modem

   c. video card

   d. CPU

5. To prevent unauthorized use of your clinic's computers, you should:

   a. establish only one person who has access to the computer

   b. keep the computer in a locked cabinet at night

   c. assign every employee a password

   d. have only one person on the computer at a time

SELF-ASSESSMENT

How comfortable are you with moving a computer from one area to another and hooking up all the cords, connections, and wires? What do you think you could do to become more comfortable with computer hardware connections? Look at the connections of your computer and its accessory hardware. Is it color coded or marked in some way?

_____

_____

_____

_____

CHAPTER **12**

Telecommunications

CHAPTER PRE-TEST

Perform this test without looking at your book. If an answer is "false," rewrite the sentence to make it true.

1. True or False? When transferring a call, it is not necessary to obtain the patient's name and phone number.

_____

_____

2. True or False? Some patients need to be handled with a firm voice on the phone.

_____

_____

3. True or False? It is not necessary to ask permission prior to putting a patient on hold.

_____

_____

4. True or False? When taking a message, be as brief as possible. The patient's name and phone number is enough information.

_____

_____

5. True or False? Patients cannot expect confidentiality on their home answering machines.

_____

_____

6. True or False? All angry calls should be immediately forwarded to the provider.

_____

_____

VOCABULARY BUILDER

Misspelled Words

Find the words below that are misspelled; circle them, and correctly spell them in the spaces provided. Then fill in the blanks in the following paragraph with the appropriate terms. (Hint: not all terms will be used.)

answering services	etiguette	jargon
articulate	faximile	modulated
buffer words	fluant	obfucation
clincial email	Good Samaritan laws	pagers
enunciate	handheld devices	pronounciation

_____   _____   _____

_____   _____   _____

When speaking on the telephone, medical assistants must use proper telephone _____, which means being courteous and professional to others. To ensure that listeners understand what is said, it is important to _____, or say the words clearly. Simple terms rather than medical _____ promote mutual understanding rather than confusion or _____. The use of slang words and expressions is considered unprofessional and disrespectful. When speaking with a caller who is not _____ in English, it is helpful to speak slowly and use short sentences. Proper _____ of all words in a carefully _____ voice will also help people understand what you are saying, especially non–English-speaking people. Good communication skills are of real benefit to a medical assistant when using the telephone and when speaking directly to patients.

Matching

Match the following devices or services listed in Column A with corresponding descriptions in Column B.

_____ 1. pager

_____ 2. answering service

_____ 3. cellular phone

_____ 4. automated routing unit

_____ 5. fax

_____ 6. email

A. Takes calls when the office is closed

B. Sends a message via phone lines to an electronic mailbox located in another person's computer

C. A one-way communication device used to contact staff when away from the office

D. A portable telephone

E. A document sent over telephone lines from one facsimile machine or modem to another

F. A system that allows callers to reach specific people or departments by pressing a specified number on a touch-tone telephone

LEARNING REVIEW

Short Answer

1. Name four reasons why a potential patient will contact an ambulatory care facility by telephone.

   _____

   _____

   _____

   _____

2. Many providers and health care professionals use paging systems. Paging systems allow the medical assistant to alert a provider or other health care professional who is not on-site to call in for an important message. Name and describe four paging system options.

   _____

   _____

   _____

   _____

   _____

   _____

   _____

3. Many hospitals and ambulatory care settings have telephone systems to manage heavy telephone traffic; these are called _____.

4. No call should be left unattended for more than _____ seconds.

5. What is the difference between enunciation and pronunciation?

   _____

   _____

6. Name the three different types of Voice-over-Internet Protocol (VoIP) services in use.

   _____

   _____

7. List three advantages of email and three disadvantages of email.
   Advantages:

   _____

   _____

   _____

   _____

   Disadvantages:

   _____

   _____

   _____

8. Explain the difference between email and clinical email.

_____

_____

_____

_____

9. Why is it important for email to be encrypted?

_____

_____

Scope of Practice Review

Indicate the calls described below that fall within the scope of practice for a medical assistant (MA) to respond to and the calls that should be directed to the provider (P).

Type of Call	Who Should Handle
Insurance questions	_____
Scheduling patient testing and office appointments	_____
Medical advice	_____
Requests for prescription refills	_____
Provider's family members	_____
General information about the practice	_____
Poor progress reports from a patient	_____
Requests for medications other than prescription refills	_____
Other providers	_____
Salespeople	_____
STAT reports	_____

Patient Confidentiality Activity

Because medical assistants must observe laws regarding both patient confidentiality and the patient's right to privacy, it is crucial for the medical assistant to understand and comply with legal and ethical principles and the restrictions governing the issues of patient confidentiality. Indicate by checking off the appropriate box whether the medical assistant may discuss a patient's medical condition or reveal details from the medical record.

	Yes	No	Yes, with signed release
Patient's spouse or family member			
Patient's employer			
Patient's attorney			
Another health care provider			
Patient's insurance carrier			
Referring provider's office			
Credit bureau or collection agency			
Member of the office staff, as necessary for patient care			
Other patient			
People outside the office (friend, family acquaintance)			
Patient's parent or legal guardian, except concerning issues of birth control, abortion, or STDs			

CERTIFICATION REVIEW

These questions are designed to mimic the certification examination. Select the best response.

1. Telephone calls that may be handled by the medical assistant include all but which one of the following?

   a. Billing questions

   b. Appointment changes

   c. Requests for prescription refills

   d. Calls from other physicians

2. When a medical assistant is talking to a patient on the telephone and another line rings, what should the medical assistant do?

   a. Ask permission from the first caller to put her on hold, answer the second call and then ask permission from that caller to put him on hold, and go back to the first caller to finish up.

   b. Put the first call on hold, answer the second call and handle that issue, then go back to the first caller.

   c. Let the second line ring; it will be picked up by an answering system.

   d. Finish with the first caller, then answer the second line.

3. Which of the following is *not* a good idea in a medical office?

   a. Using a speaker phone to listen to voice messages

   b. Speaking quietly on the telephone so other patients cannot hear

   c. Using a privacy screen to reduce the chance of being overheard on the telephone

   d. Using only email so you will not be overheard

4. After-hours telephone messages are usually directed to:

   a. the provider's home

   b. the medical manager's home

   c. a voice mail system or answering service/machine

   d. an email system

5. When talking to older adult patients on the phone:

   a. if the patient is hearing impaired, speak slower, clearer, and a little louder

   b. assume that they are senile or at least forgetful and repeat all the information several times

   c. if the person has difficulty understanding, simplify the information, ask if there are any questions, and try to explain patiently in simple terms

   d. All of the above

   e. a. and c. only

6. Guidelines of the Health Insurance Portability and Accountability Act (HIPAA) for telephone communication include:

   a. Determine if patients have specific instructions on who has been granted privilege to their private medical information.

   b. Determine if patients have a particular number they want called for confidential communications.

   c. Ask if it is acceptable to leave a message if patients are not at the number provided.

   d. All of the above

7. The best solution for handling a caller who refuses to give information after gentle prodding is:

   a. tell the patient to call back when he is ready to cooperate

   b. hang up on the caller

   c. take a message and then give it to the provider

   d. argue with the patient, telling him that he is being unreasonable and that you need the information

8. The administrative medical assistant should always try to answer a call:

   a. by the end of the first ring if possible but definitely within three rings

   b. after five rings

   c. after two rings and before five rings

   d. within a minute

9. Before transferring a call to the appropriate party, a guideline to follow is:

   a. Put the caller on hold, then transfer the call.

   b. Put the caller on hold and contact the person to whom the call is going, to see if the person can speak to the caller.

   c. Transfer the call immediately.

   d. Get the caller's name, number, and any pertinent information.

10. If a call is a medical emergency, what protocol should be followed in handling that type of situation?

   a. Tell the patient to go to the emergency room.

   b. Keep the caller on the line and call 911 on another line.

   c. Put the caller on hold and try to get the provider on the phone.

   d. Tell the patient that you will call 911 for her and then call her back.

11. To ensure sensible risk management when making calls, you should protect the patient's privacy at all times; this is referred to as:

   a. confidentiality

   b. jargon

   c. elaboration

   d. screening

LEARNING APPLICATION

 CASE STUDY

As Inner City Health Care, an urgent care center, continues to grow, increasing both patient load and staff, the existing telephone system, consisting of a simple intercom and four telephone lines, is no longer sufficient to handle the call volume and allow for full, immediate accessibility for all staff members. Callers are frustrated by the length of time it takes to get through and by long amounts of time spent on hold. Messages are often late in getting properly routed. Administrative medical assistant Karen Ritter suggests to office manager Jane O'Hara that an automated routing unit (ARU) might be more efficient for the growing clinic's needs. At the next regularly scheduled staff meeting, the provider-employers give the go-ahead to research an ARU.

CASE STUDY REVIEW QUESTIONS

1. ARU systems provide several options for callers that identify specific departments or services that callers can be connected with directly. What kinds of caller options might be appropriate for Inner City Health Care?

   _____

   _____

   _____

   _____

   _____

   _____

2. What can be done so the patient with an emergency or the hearing-impaired patient can speak automatically to a "live" operator?

   _____

   _____

   _____

   _____

continues

3. How can an ARU help staff members receive their calls more efficiently?

_____

_____

_____

4. How can the office manager and medical assistant implement the ARU system with a minimum of disruption to provider(s), staff, and patients?

_____

_____

_____

_____

_____

_____

Role-Play Exercises

Effective telephone communication requires prompt and professional responses from medical assistants. With another student, role-play as patient and medical assistant. When you are finished role-playing, write what you have said as the "medical assistant" below.

1. Patient Nora Fowler calls with a question about medication prescribed for her rheumatoid arthritis and insists on a call back from Dr. Elizabeth King. Dr. King is presently on rounds at the hospital and will not be available until 4:30 PM. Nora's tone of voice indicates that she is upset, and she states that her medication is not helping her discomfort. It is clear from the conversation that Nora has discontinued taking her medication.

_____

_____

_____

_____

_____

_____

2. While speaking on telephone line 1 with patient Bill Schwartz, who is calling to schedule a physical examination, medical assistant Wanda Slawson receives another call on line 2 from a laboratory with a summary of emergency test results for another patient. Wanda knows that Dr. Susan Rice is waiting for the test results.

_____

_____

_____

_____

3. Medical assistant Bruce Goldman takes a call from patient Juanita Hansen. Juanita is inquiring about a bill and indicating that her insurance carrier, Blue Cross, did not pay the entire fee for her son's last examination, which left her with a balance owed to Inner City Health Care. Office manager Walter Seals is responsible for managing insurance claims and inquiries.

_____

_____

_____

Hands-on Activities

1. Each morning, medical assistant Ellen Armstrong is responsible for transcribing messages left on the medical practice's answering machine the evening before. Using the message pad slips below, transcribe each message completely and appropriately. In the space for "Attachments," list any records, files, or documents that should be attached to the message slip for the recipient's review.

   A. "Ellen, this is Anna Preciado. Can you tell Marilyn Johnson, the office manager, that I won't be in tomorrow for the afternoon shift? I have a 101-degree temperature and bad flu symptoms. Check with Joe Guerrero to see if he can come in to sub for me as the clinical medical assistant. Yesterday he told me he would be available if I wasn't feeling well enough to come in. I know Dr. Lewis has several patients scheduled for clinical testing in the afternoon. I can be reached at 555-6622."

   B. "This is Charles Williams. Dr. Lewis put me on a Holter monitor today. It's about 11:00 PM and one of the leads came off. I put it back on, but I am worried about whether I will have to do this test again. Can you call me tomorrow at home before 8:00 AM at 555-6124 or at the office after 9:00 AM at 555-8125? Thanks."

To: _____ Date: _____
From: _____ Time: _____
Telephone #: _____

Message: _____
_____
_____
_____
Initials: _____
Attachments: _____
_____

To: _____ Date: _____
From: _____ Time: _____
Telephone #: _____

Message: _____
_____
_____
_____
Initials: _____
Attachments: _____
_____

CHAPTER POST-TEST

Perform this test without looking at your book. If an answer is "false," rewrite the sentence to make it true.

1. True or False? When transferring a call, it is important to obtain the patient's name and phone number.

_____

_____

2. True or False? Some patients will become defensive when a firm voice is used on the phone.

_____

_____

3. True or False? The patient should always be asked if she can be put on hold.

_____

_____

4. True or False? When taking a message, be brief but thorough. The patient's name, phone number, questions, best time for a callback, and any other pertinent information that is useful should be noted.

_____

_____

5. True or False? Patients should expect confidentiality at all times, even on their home answering machines.

_____

_____

6. True or False? The provider should be alerted to any angry calls regarding patient care and treatment.

_____

_____

SELF-ASSESSMENT

1. Discuss the following questions with another classmate or in a small group. During the discussion, consider how different people react in different ways, depending on their personalities, their patience, and their confidence levels. After the discussion, spend a moment in self-reflection to think of ways you can improve your telephone communication skills.

   (1) Have you ever conversed with someone on the telephone whom you could not understand?

   _____

   _____

   (2) Was it the language of the individual, their accent, enunciation, or volume?

   _____

   _____

   (3) Would it have been easier to understand the individual if you were face to face with that person?

   _____

   _____

(4) How did you handle the situation? Did you ask the person to speak louder, slower, or more clearly?

_____

_____

(5) How do you think most people would handle a situation in which they could not hear the speaker clearly? What if the speaker were an older adult? a non–English speaker? A person in pain or very ill?

_____

_____

2. Of the following telecommunication devices and methods, with which are you most familiar and which will you need to learn more about? What do you think is the best way to become more familiar with the following devices and methods?
   - Email
   - Pagers
   - Multiline phones
   - Cell phones
   - Fax machines
   - Answering services

_____

_____

_____

_____

C H A P T E R **13**

Patient Scheduling

CHAPTER PRE-TEST

Perform this test without looking at your book. If an answer is "false," rewrite the sentence to make it true.

1. Circle the letter that lists correct types of scheduling systems:

   a. wave, modified wave, double booking, mile-a-minute

   b. open hours, wave, clustering, stream, double booking

   c. first-come, first-served; open hours; clustering

2. Below are guidelines to scheduling. Which one is correct?

   a. Urgent calls should be sent to the hospital, which is better equipped to handle them.

   b. Urgent calls should be assessed before determining the best course of action.

   c. Referrals by other physicians need to be seen immediately.

   d. Appointments for pharmaceutical and medical supply representatives should be referred to the physician.

3. Information that should be obtained from all new patients includes all but which one of the following?

   a. The patient's full legal name

   b. The patient's birth date

   c. The patient's address and telephone numbers

   d. The reason for the visit

   e. The patient's insurance information

   f. The patient's family health history

4. True or False? All medical offices are changing to electronic appointment scheduling.

   _____

   _____

5. True or False? When providing a sign-in sheet for patients, it is permissible to request the reason for the visit.

   _____

   _____

6. True or False? It is not necessary to note cancellations or no-shows in the patient's chart.

_____

_____

VOCABULARY BUILDER

Misspelled Words

Find the words below that are misspelled; circle them, and correctly spell them in the spaces provided. Then replace the highlighted words in the following paragraph with the correct vocabulary terms from the list.

clustering	modified wave scheduling	screaning
double booking	no-show	stream scheduling
encription technology	open hours	wave scheduling
matrics	practice based	

_____   _____   _____

_____

1. Inner City Health Care reserves 9 AM to 12 PM on Thursday mornings for walk-in patients who are seen on a first-come, first-served basis within that time frame.

_____

2. At the offices of Drs. Lewis and King, Ellen Armstrong, CMA (AAMA), schedules Mary O'Keefe for a 1:00 PM appointment for some blood work and Martin Gordon for a 1:00 PM appointment for a blood pressure check so Dr. King can assess whether his medication is at the proper level.

_____

3. Lenny Taylor, an older adult patient with mild dementia, forgets his third appointment with Dr. James Whitney.

_____

4. At Inner City Health Care, vaccinations are scheduled every 10 minutes from 10 AM to 12:20 PM on Mondays; Tuesday office hours are reserved for new patients only.

_____

5. Three patients are scheduled to receive treatments in the first half hour of every hour.

_____

6. Dr. Elizabeth King prefers to see patients for regular gynecologic examinations in consecutive appointments scheduled from 8:30 AM to 11:30 AM and obstetric patients from 1:00 PM to 3:30 PM.

_____

7. When patient Herb Fowler calls to set up an appointment with Dr. Winston Lewis for his chronic cough, Ellen Armstrong, CMA (AAMA), asks Herb a series of questions to ascertain the nature, extent, and urgency of his condition.

_____

8. Dr. Winston Lewis prefers that each patient be assigned a specific time, scheduling at 30- or 60-minute intervals on a continuous basis throughout the day.

_____

9. An ophthalmologist schedules three patients at the beginning of each hour for comprehensive examinations, followed by single appointments every 10 to 20 minutes during the rest of the hour for quick, follow-up procedures such as removing eye patches or instilling eye drops.

_____

10. On the 15th day of each month, office manager Walter Seals, who is responsible for efficient patient flow at Inner City Health Care, asks each of the urgent care center's five providers to confirm their scheduling commitments for the upcoming month to block off unavailable times in the appointment book.

_____

11. The medical assistant uses software to protect patients' confidentiality in electronic format.

LEARNING REVIEW

Short Answer

1. Appointment books are legal documents recording patient flow. For a manual appointment system, where pencil is used for ease in rescheduling, what can the medical assistant do to ensure that a permanent record is secured?

   _____

   _____

   _____

2. For a computerized appointment system, what can a medical assistant do to ensure that a permanent record of patient flow is secured?

   _____

   _____

   _____

   _____

3. Name two primary goals in determining the best method for scheduling patient appointments.

   _____

   _____

   _____

4. What is the typical scheduling time for each of the following types of office visits for an internal medicine practice?

   (1) Patient consultation: _____

   (2) Established patient routine follow-up: _____

   (3) New patient: _____

   (4) Complete physical examination: _____

   (5) Cold/flu symptoms: _____

   (6) Vaccination: _____

5. What are six variables involved in the process of scheduling appointments for patients and other visitors to the ambulatory care setting?

   _____

   _____

   _____

   _____

   _____

6. Patient flow analysis sheets help medical practices determine the effectiveness of patient scheduling and devise plans for improving a smooth patient flow through the ambulatory care setting. What kinds of issues can a study of these data reveal?

   _____

   _____

   _____

7. What are the five steps of scheduling a specific appointment time for a patient?

_____

_____

_____

_____

_____

_____

8. Two ways of reminding patients of upcoming appointments are to give the appointment card personally to the patient and to mail the card to the patient. Identify a third reminder system. What procedures must be observed to protect patient confidentiality when using this third method?

_____

_____

_____

_____

9. Identify seven scheduling styles.

_____

_____

10. Identify the best scheduling system for the examples below, and explain the reasoning behind your choice.
   (1) Hospital emergency room:

   _____

   _____

   _____

   _____

   (2) Laboratory for blood testing:

   _____

   _____

   _____

   _____

   (3) Two or more patients are given a particular appointment time:

   _____

   _____

   (4) Best-known and widely used scheduling system:

   _____

   _____

   _____

11. Patient Mark Johnson is a no-show for his appointment. Other than marking the no-show appropriately on the appointment schedule, what other action must be taken to document Mr. Johnson's no-show status? Why is it important to accurately and completely document patient no-shows and cancellations?

_____

_____

_____

_____

_____

_____

_____

True or False

Mark a true statement with a T *and a false statement with an* F. *If an answer is "false," rewrite the sentence to make it true.*

____ 1. In scheduling, double booking means to keep two appointment books going for the same doctor.

_____

_____

____ 2. One major purpose of screening when scheduling appointments is to determine if the patient has an emergency or urgent situation/illness.

_____

_____

____ 3. If a patient routinely cancels or misses three consecutive appointments, the provider may decide to terminate services.

_____

_____

____ 4. The appointment book/record may be subpoenaed, and therefore is considered a legal document.

_____

_____

____ 5. Providing patients with appointment cards is an effective way to prevent missed appointments.

_____

_____

____ 6. It is important to provide an appointment to a referral patient as soon as possible.

_____

_____

____ 7. There is an unexpected delay in the schedule caused by an office emergency. It is not necessary for the medical assistant to provide the patient with an estimate of how long the delay will be.

_____

_____

____ 8. A hurried, disinterested manner toward patients is just as often the basis for legal action as is a negligent act.

_____

_____

____ 9. A permanent record or daily appointment sheet does not have to indicate any changes such as cancellations, walk-ins, urgent care needs, and no-shows.

_____

_____

____ 10. If at the same time when scheduling an appointment for a patient in the office, the phone rings, the medical assistant should first excuse herself and take the call.

_____

_____

CERTIFICATION REVIEW

These questions are designed to mimic the certification examination. Select the best response.

1. Scheduling outpatient procedures:

   a. is done at the end of each day

   b. is best done with the patient present

   c. will be easier with a calendar for visualization of days discussed

   d. b. and c.

2. One principle above all else in scheduling for the office is:

   a. flexibility

   b. neatness

   c. accountability

   d. estimation

3. The type of scheduling that requires visits to be set up around patients with specific chronic ailments such as diabetes and hypertension is called:

   a. screening

   b. referral appointments

   c. group scheduling

   d. stream appointments

4. The general rule for no-shows and cancellations is that after _____ consecutive missed appointments, the provider will review the patient's record and could terminate care.

   a. five

   b. three

   c. two

   d. ten

5. What, more than anything else, determines the success of a day in the ambulatory care setting?

   a. Patient care

   b. Efficient patient flow

   c. Operational functions

   d. Interpersonal skills

LEARNING APPLICATION

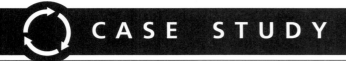

CASE STUDY

When patient Lenore McDonell falls from the examination table and lacerates her arm while attempting an independent transfer from the table to her wheelchair, clinical medical assistant Joe Guerrero alerts Dr. Winston Lewis, and the two begin to implement emergency procedures to control Lenore's bleeding and assess damage to the arm. Lenore's fall occurred at the end of her appointment, a routine checkup with Dr. Lewis.

Administrative medial assistant Ellen Armstrong must adjust Dr. Lewis's schedule to accommodate the emergency situation. Martin Gordon, a man in his mid-60s, diagnosed with prostate cancer, waits in the reception area for Dr. Lewis's next appointment. Mr. Gordon's appointment, a 6-month follow-up, is expected to take 30 minutes. Mr. Gordon is also being rated for depression related to his cancer diagnosis. Hope Smith, a new patient in good general health, is scheduled for a complete examination; she is due to arrive at the office of Drs. Lewis and King at the Northborough Family Medical Group within 20 minutes. Jim Marshall, an impatient and aggressive businessman, is scheduled for the first afternoon appointment after Dr. Lewis's lunch commitment. Mr. Marshall's appointment for a physical examination and ECG to investigate chest pains he has experienced recently is expected to take 45 minutes. Dr. Lewis's schedule is completely booked for the rest of the day.

CASE STUDY REVIEW QUESTIONS

1. What scheduling alternatives will Ellen offer Mr. Gordon, who is already waiting in the reception area? What special considerations regarding Mr. Gordon should Ellen take into account and why?

    _____

    _____

    _____

    _____

    _____

    _____

    _____

    _____

    _____

2. What is Ellen's first action regarding Ms. Smith, Dr. Lewis's next patient due to arrive? What scheduling alternatives should Ellen offer her?

    _____

    _____

    _____

    _____

    _____

    _____

continues

3. What scheduling alternatives, if any, should Ellen present to Mr. Marshall? Explain your logic.

    _____

    _____

    _____

    _____

    _____

4. How is screening important to Ellen's rescheduling of Dr. Lewis's patients? What important administrative and communication skills will Ellen use to handle this emergency situation efficiently and professionally?

    _____

    _____

    _____

    _____

    _____

    _____

    _____

    _____

    _____

    _____

    _____

Hands-on Activity

Patient Martin Gordon has a 30-minute appointment scheduled with Dr. Lewis on Wednesday, February 7, 20XX for routine follow-up for prostate cancer. He calls the office on January 30 and would like to reschedule his appointment for two weeks later at 3:00 PM the same time. You mark through his name on the appointment schedule with a single line in red pen, and document the change in the patient's chart. Now, complete the appointment card below to be mailed to Mr. Gordon as a reminder of his new appointment time.

LEWIS & KING, MD
L&K
2501 CENTER STREET
NORTHBOROUGH, OH 12345

M _____

has an appointment on

Mon. _____ at _____

Tues. _____ at _____

Wed. _____ at _____

Thurs. _____ at _____

Fri. _____ at _____

If unable to keep appointment, kindly give 24 hours' notice.

MOSS Activities

Using Medical Office Simulation Software and the skills learned in Procedure 13-4, schedule the following appointments:

1. A 30-minute appointment for Edward Gormann on July 10, 2009, for an earache.

2. A 15-minute appointment for Megan Caldwell on July 15, 2009, to check for strep throat.

CHAPTER POST-TEST

Perform this test without looking at your book. If an answer is "false," rewrite the sentence to make it true.

1. Circle the letter that lists correct types of scheduling systems.

   a. Modified wave, wave, clustering, and mile-a-minute

   b. Stream, open hours, wave, grouping, separating

   c. First-come, first-served; open hours; clustering

   d. Open hours, wave, clustering, stream, double booking

2. Below are guidelines to scheduling. Which one is correct?

   a. Urgent calls should be scheduled for the next available appointment time.

   b. Urgent calls should be sent to the hospital, which is better equipped to handle them.

   c. If a referral patient calls, it is best to obtain information from the referring provider's office to determine the urgency of the appointment.

   d. Appointments for pharmaceutical and medical supply representatives should be referred to the physician.

3. Information that should be obtained from all new patients includes all but which one of the following?

   a. The patient's full legal name

   b. The patient's birth date

   c. The patient's address and telephone numbers

   d. Family health history

   e. Reason for the visit

   f. The patient's insurance information

4. True or False? Many medical offices are changing to electronic appointment scheduling.

   _____

   _____

5. True or False? When a patient cancels or is a no-show, it must always be documented in the patient chart.

   _____

   _____

SELF-ASSESSMENT

1. When you call a provider's office, do any of the following aggravate you? Do you think other people are aggravated by these?

   a. Being put on hold right away or too often

   b. The administrative medical assistant asking too many questions

   c. Not enough appointment time choices; that is, you have to wait too long for an appointment

   d. Not getting a real person; that is, having to listen to electronic choices and make selections

   e. Other (add your own idea) _____

2. Now go to each of the situations in Question 1 and determine an action that could alleviate all or some of the aggravation. Keep in mind that the situation might still exist (e.g., the receptionist might still have to ask a lot of questions), but how might he or she make the experience more pleasant?

   _____

   _____

   _____

   _____

3. When you visit a provider's office, do any of the following aggravate you?

   a. The administrative medical assistant does not acknowledge you right away.

   b. The wait is too long.

   c. The waiting room is noisy, messy, or uncomfortable.

   d. There are no magazines of interest to you.

   e. Other (add your own idea) _____

4. Similar to the instructions in Question 2, go to each of the situations in Question 3 and determine solutions that could alleviate all or some of the causes of aggravation. Keep in mind that the solutions in this case are obvious and doable.

   _____

   _____

   _____

   _____

5. Think of your most pleasant interaction with a provider's office as a patient making an appointment, scheduling a procedure, changing an appointment, or even canceling an appointment. What made the experience more pleasant? Was it the voice of the administrative medical assistant? his or her tone? actual words? the overall options? or something else?

   _____

   _____

   _____

   _____

6. As you enter your career as a medical assistant, try to remember how the patient feels. Try to recall situations that bother you when you are a patient. Try to keep these issues in mind and see if you can eliminate or alleviate them to make your patients as comfortable as possible. Maybe you are just the person who will help to make the experience of seeing a doctor more pleasant for your patients. Try to be like the person you thought of for Question 5. This is not an easy thing to do when you are busy and stressed. Can you think of ways you can remind yourself every day of these lessons?

_____

_____

_____

_____

CHAPTER **14**

Medical Records Management

CHAPTER PRE-TEST

Perform this test without looking at your book. If an answer is "false," rewrite the sentence to make it true.

1. True or False? Out-guides indicate when patient charts are out of order.

   _____

   _____

2. Which of the following is *not* an important skill to have when filing?
   a. You should know the alphabet.

   b. You should know the basic rules of filing.

   c. You should pay attention to details.

   d. You should be good at math.

3. True or False? Medical records are important for many reasons. They provide information for medical care, legal protection, and research purposes.

   _____

   _____

4. True or False? It is acceptable to release medical information to family members as long as they can show proper picture identification.

   _____

   _____

5. True or False? The standard in court is that if there is no record of information related to the appointment, including care and treatment of that patient, then it did not happen.

   _____

   _____

6. True or False? All medical filing systems use the alphabetic filing system.

   _____

   _____

VOCABULARY BUILDER

Misspelled Words

Find the words below that are misspelled; underline them, and correctly spell them in the space provided. Then, fill in the blanks in the following sentences with the appropriate terms. (Hint: not all words will be used.)

accession record	key unit	SOAP
captions	out-gide	source-orientated medical record
coding	perging	tickler file
cross-reference	problem-orientated medical record	unit

_____   _____   _____

_____

1. To remember to check with the reference laboratory on Friday to obtain patient Martin Gordon's test results, Ellen Armstrong, CMA (AAMA), places a note in her _____.

2. Every six months, Marilyn Johnson follows office policy and procedures for _____ inactive files to remove and archive those not in active use.

3. The organized method of identifying and separating items to be filed into small subunits is accomplished with the use of _____ units.

4. When Liz Corbin, CMA (AAMA), retrieves Annette Samuels's chart for Dr. Woo, she places an _____ in the filing cabinet to show that the file has been removed from storage.

5. The _____ is a journal (or computer listing) where numbers in a numeric filing system are pre-assigned. The log sequentially lists numbers to be used to assign to numeric records.

6. The file for Kent Memorial Hospital contains three indexing _____ to be considered when preparing the filing label.

7. If a _____ card is required in the alphabetic card file of a numeric filing system, such as when making note of an established patient's married name, a card is prepared that includes an **X** next to the file number to indicate that this card does not designate the primary location card for the file.

8. In the _____ system of recordkeeping, patient problems are identified by a number that corresponds to the charting relevant to that problem number; that is, asthma #1; dermatitis #2; and so on.

9. When a filing system other than alphabetic is being used, the proper _____ must be determined for the chart or file so it can be retrieved.

10. _____ are used to identify major sections of file folders by more manageable subunits, such as GA-GE, or Miscellaneous. Captions are marked on the tabs of the guides.

11. Inner City Health Care uses the _____ method of recordkeeping, which groups information according to its origin; for example, laboratories, examinations, provider notes, consulting providers, and other types of information.

12. Some medical facilities have added two additional letters, "E" and "R," to the _____ approach, which stand for "education for patient" and "response of patient to education and care given."

LEARNING REVIEW

Short Answer

1. Why is accurate, up-to-date, complete documentation in patient medical records essential in the ambulatory care setting?

   _____

   _____

   _____

   _____

   _____

2. Why is the POMR system commonly used by family practice offices?

   _____

   _____

   _____

3. Why is a color-coding system effective in the ambulatory care setting?

   _____

   _____

4. How important is an effective, easy-to-use, and easy-to-access filing system to the efficiency of the ambulatory care setting?

   _____

   _____

   _____

   _____

   _____

   _____

5. List at least four advantages of EMRs.

   _____

   _____

   _____

   _____

6. What does the acronym SOAPER stand for?

   _____

   _____

   _____

7. List three numeric filing systems that are used in medical facilities.

   _____

   _____

8. List at least five standards required by the HIPAA Security Rule for electronic medical records.

_____

_____

_____

_____

_____

_____

_____

Indexing Units Exercise

Assign the correct units to the following items to be filed using the rule for filing patient records that is listed for each.

1. Names that are hyphenated are considered one unit.

   A. Jackson Hugh Levine-Dwyer

   unit 1 _____ unit 2 _____ unit 3 _____

   B. Leslie Jane Poole-Petit

   unit 1 _____ unit 2 _____ unit 3 _____

2. Seniority units are indexed as the last indexing unit.

   A. Keith Wildasin Sr.

   unit 1 _____ unit 2 _____ unit 3 _____

   B. Gerald Maggart III

   unit 1 _____ unit 2 _____ unit 3 _____

3. Titles are considered as separate indexing units. If the title appears with first and last names, the title is considered the last indexing unit.

   A. Dr. Louise Udolf

   unit 1 _____ unit 2 _____ unit 3 _____

   B. Prof. Valerie Rajah

   unit 1 _____ unit 2 _____ unit 3 _____

4. The names of individuals are assigned indexing units respectively: last name, first name, middle, and succeeding names.

   A. Lindsay Adair Martin

   unit 1 _____ unit 2 _____ unit 3 _____

   B. Abigail Sue Johnson

   unit 1 _____ unit 2 _____ unit 3 _____

5. When indexing names of married women, the name is indexed by the legal name.

   A. Mary Jane O'Keefe (Mrs. John)

   unit 1 _____ unit 2 _____ unit 3 _____ unit 4 _____

   B. Nora Patrice Fowler (Mrs. Herb)

   unit 1 _____ unit 2 _____ unit 3 _____ unit 4 _____

6. Foreign language units are indexed as one unit with the unit that follows. Spacing, punctuation, and capitalization are ignored.

   A. Joseph Jack de la Hoya

   unit 1 _____ unit 2 _____ unit 3 _____

   B. Maurice John van de Veer

   unit 1 _____ unit 2 _____ unit 3 _____

Multiple Choice

Circle the right answer(s) from the choices below.

1. The most important reason for using numeric filing is that:
   a. it preserves patient confidentiality
   b. a larger number of records can be easily filed
   c. a computer can more readily read numeric filing labels

2. Walter Seals, CMA (AAMA), is filing using a terminal digit filing system. For the patient file labeled 67 84 30, what is unit 1?
   a. 67
   b. 30
   c. 80

3. Outgoing correspondence is:
   a. friendly correspondence
   b. correspondence sent out of the medical office
   c. correspondence to be thrown away

4. Karen Ritter, CMA (AAMA), is filing patient files using a numeric filing system. She comes across a file for a patient who has not yet been assigned a number. Karen should put the file:
   a. in the miscellaneous numeric file section
   b. in a pending filing bin until the provider can assign a number
   c. directly behind the rest of the files

5. An out-guide in paper or manual records should contain:
   a. a record of when the chart was removed
   b. the signature of the patient's physician
   c. a record of when the file is expected to be returned

6. State statutes have ruled that medical records are the property of the:
   a. state medical society
   b. ones who create them
   c. patient only

7. Any information to be released from the medical record:
   a. goes to medical insurance
   b. requires a provider's signature
   c. requires patient notification and approval
   d. requires a subpoena

8. Filing equipment:
   a. should have a locking capability

   b. is available in vertical or lateral styles

   c. is to be stored in an area accessible only to authorized personnel

   d. All of the above

9. EMR stands for:
   a. emergency room

   b. a popular color-coding system's trade name

   c. electronic medical records

   d. emergency medical rules

10. Release marks include:
    a. date stamp and initials

    b. out-guides

    c. tabs

    d. SOAP/SOAPER

CERTIFICATION REVIEW

These questions are designed to mimic the certification examination. Select the best response.

1. The POMR is also known as:

   a. a source-oriented medical record

   b. a SOAP/SOAPER system

   c. a traditional method

   d. a problem-oriented medical record

   e. none of the above

2. The SOAP/SOAPER format is:

   a. a way to sanitize instruments

   b. a form of patient electronic records

   c. a type of filing system

   d. a specific charting system

   e. none of the above

3. If a patient needs to return for another examination in six months, you might use a reminder system. What is the name of that system?

   a. Reminder system

   b. Recall system

   c. Phone log

   d. Tickler system

   e. Out-guide

4. The most common method of filing in today's medical office is:

   a. alphabetically

   b. numerically

   c. by insurance

   d. by subject

   e. color coding

5. If a medical document is filed in multiple places, you might use a(n):

   a. index

   b. out-guide

   c. cross-reference

   d. multiple reference

   e. cross-filed card

6. The best method to use for making a correction in a paper medical record is:

   a. use a "white out" product

   b. scribble over the error with a magic marker

   c. put "x's" through the error

   d. draw a single line through the error, make the correction, write "CORR" or "CORRECTION" above the area corrected, and add your initials and date.

7. Identifiable patient information that should *not* appear on the outside of the chart would include:

   a. patient's address

   b. patient's social security number

   c. patient's birth date

   d. patient's phone number

   e. all of the above

8. Closed files are usually kept:

   a. 3 to 6 years beyond the statute of limitations

   b. 2 to 5 years

   c. indefinitely

   d. 10 years

9. The three types of cabinets used in medical clinics are:

   a. vertical, lateral, and movable

   b. metal, hanging, and color coded

   c. horizontal, lateral, and movable

   d. open, locked, and movable

10. Captions are used:

   a. to separate file folders

   b. to identify major sections of file folders

   c. in vertical and lateral systems

   d. a. and c. only

LEARNING APPLICATION

Filing Order Review

Using the numbers 1, 2, and 3, label the patient names in each group according to the correct filing order of names in an alphabetic filing system.

____ L. Sanders

____ Larry Paul Samuels

____ Lawrence P. Sanders

____ James Edward Reed Sr.

____ James Edward Reed

____ James Edward Reed Jr.

____ Lynn Elaine Brenner

____ Lynn Ellen Brenner

____ Lynn Eloise Brenner

____ Patrick Sam Saint

____ Patrick Sam St. Bartz

____ Paul Sam Saint

MOSS Activities

Using Medical Office Simulation Software and the skills learned in Procedure 14-7, register the following new patients, to establish a new record for each.

1. Ms. Julia E. Martin, a new patient of Dr. Schwartz. (Hint: Dr. Schwartz is a participating provider of Julia's insurance plan, ConsumerOne HRA, and accepts assignment.)

Home contact information	13 Cobble Stone Ave Douglasville, NY 01234 (123) 457-1212
Marital Status	Single
Social Security Number	999-76-1234
Date of Birth	December 1, 1980
Employer	Clear Lake Elementary 5526 Gravel Way, Douglasville, NY 01234 (123) 528-1132
Primary Insurance Information	ConsumerOne HRA ID Number: 999761234-01 Group Number: CLE5610 Policyholder: Self

2. Mr. Adair Smith, a new patient of Dr. Heath, who was referred by Dr. Samantha Green. (Hint: Dr. Heath is a participating provider of Adair's insurance plan, Medicare, and accepts assignment.)

Home contact information	159 Broad Street Douglasville, NY 01234 (123) 528-4092
Marital Status	Married to Mackenzie Smith
Social Security Number	999-54-3579
Date of Birth	April 26, 1938
Employer	Retired
Primary Insurance Information	Medicare ID Number: 999543579A

3. Remi Beaufort, a new patient of Dr. Heath, who is brought to the office by his father, Joseph Beaufort. (Hint: Dr. Heath is a participating provider of the insurance plan, and accepts assignment.)

Home contact information	43 Clay Lane Douglasville, NY 01234 (123) 457-3393
Marital Status	Single
Social Security Number	999-23-8989
Date of Birth	June 8, 1991
Employer	Full-time student at Clear Lake Elementary
Guarantor information	Joseph Beaufort Social Security Number: 999-44-8754 Date of Birth: August 17, 1964 Employer: The Rockwell Group
Primary Insurance Information	Signal HMO Policyholder: Joseph Beaufort ID Number: 999448754-03 Group Number: TRG01 Office co-pay: $10.00

CHAPTER POST-TEST

Perform this test without looking at your book. If an answer is "false," rewrite the sentence to make it true.

1. True or False? When patient charts are out of order, we use out-guides to help us see the error better.

_____

_____

2. When filing, you need to be skilled in all but which one of the following?

   a. Knowing the alphabet

   b. Knowing the basic rules of filing

   c. Being able to pay attention to details

   d. Being good at math

3. True or False? Medical records are important for many reasons. Their most important purpose is for legal protection.

   _____

   _____

4. True or False? It is acceptable to release medical information to a family member as long as you have written authorization from the patient.

   _____

   _____

5. True or False? Proper documentation in a patient's chart is the standard in court because if there is no record of treatment, then it did not happen.

   _____

   _____

6. True or False? Medical filing systems may be based on the alphabet, a numeric system, or by subject.

   _____

   _____

SELF-ASSESSMENT

To perform this self-assessment, you must first perform an exercise: Go to your spice drawer, a stack of magazines, a bunch of bills/statements, or even your clothes closet, drawers, or the shelves you keep your towels on. (Maybe organize something in your medical assisting classroom or laboratory area!)

1. Think of the best way to organize them. Is it by size, color, or both? Alphabetically? By date? Frequency of use?

   _____

   _____

   _____

2. Perform the organization. What was the most difficult part: planning how to best accomplish it, or actually doing it? Did you have to take everything out and place it back in order, or were you able to just move things around? Was this a time-consuming exercise? Is the order now a useful tool? Did you have any decisions to make, such as do you file red pepper under red or pepper? Should your pants be organized with their matching tops, or should all the pants be together and all the tops together? Should the medications be organized in alphabetic order, or by classification (type of action)?

   _____

   _____

   _____

   _____

3. Now choose another item to organize in a different way. How did this second exercise differ? (For example, towels might have been organized by size or by color, whereas your spices would be organized alphabetically.) Do you think another person would have chosen a different method?

_____

_____

_____

_____

4. Who do you think decides in an office how a particular area is to be organized? Do you think there might be different ways?

_____

_____

_____

_____

5. Pretend that your provider's office has its patients' charts filed alphabetically, but now they are moving to more computerized records and want to change their files to a numeric system. Make a list of the supplies the staff will need, calculate the time it might take, and make up a plan on how to accomplish this (remember the files are still being used every day). Does this seem like a major undertaking? Could any files be purged (pulled out of circulation) during this reorganization?

_____

_____

_____

_____

C H A P T E R **15**

Written Communications

CHAPTER PRE-TEST

Perform this test without looking at your book. If an answer is "false," rewrite the sentence to make it true.

1. The four major letter styles are *(circle four of the following):*

   a. full block

   b. modified block, standard

   c. facilitated block

   d. simplified block

   e. simplified

   f. modified block, indented

2. The part of a letter that includes a specially designed logo with the address and phone numbers is called the:

   a. salutation

   b. inside address

   c. letterhead

   d. reference heading

   e. enclosure

3. True or False? Whenever documents are to be included in a mailed letter, the word *enclosure* should be written out completely and placed one or two lines below the reference initials.

   _____

   _____

4. True or False? Envelopes should be addressed using block (uppercase) letters and no punctuation.

   _____

   _____

5. A computerized feature that allows you to send the same letter, although personalized, to many different people using a database is called:

   a. word processing letters

   b. mail merge

   c. database letters

   d. merge correspondence

6. True or False? All letters in the complimentary closure are uppercase.

_____

_____

VOCABULARY BUILDER

Misspelled Words

Find the words below that are misspelled; underline them, and correctly spell them in the space provided. Then, fill in the blanks in the passage below with the correct vocabulary terms. (Hint: not all terms will be used.)

bond paper	mail merge	proofread
form letters	modified block letter	simplified letter
full block letter	optical character reader	watermarque
keed	portfoleo	ZIP+4

_____   _____   _____

There are four major types of letter styles in which medical assistants commonly write. Of these, the _____ _____ style is the most time-efficient, because it does not use excessive tab indentations for the address, complimentary closure, or keyed signature. In the _____ style, all lines begin at the left margin with the exception of the date line, complimentary closure, and keyed signature. Medical assistants may choose to use the _____ style, which is the style of letter recommended by the Administrative Management Society. In this style, all lines are _____, or input by keystroke, flush with the left margin. When selecting paper supplies, the medical assistant should choose _____ with a _____, or image imprinted during the papermaking process that is visible when a sheet is held up to the light. When preparing letters for outgoing shipments, it is important for the medical assistant to pay attention to several factors, including addresses. Medical assistants should machine-print addresses (including the _____ code) with a uniform left-hand margin so that the addresses can be read by the U.S. Postal Service's _____ (abbreviated OCR). One creative approach to letter composition is to create a _____ or database of frequently used _____.

LEARNING REVIEW

Abbreviations Exercise

Write what each abbreviation stands for.

1. Enc.   _____

2. c   _____

3. P.S.   _____

4. OCR   _____

5. CAP   _____

6. ROM   _____

7. LC   _____

8. WF   _____

Matching

Match the common proofreader's mark in Column I to its meaning in Column II.

____ 1. #   A. "Let it stand"

____ 2. ^   B. Paragraph indent

____ 3. BF   C. Insert space

____ 4. STET   D. Move left

____ 5.]   E. Italic type

____ 6. [F. Align type horizontally

____ 7. :| G. Insert

____ 8. =   H. Boldface type

____ 9. ITAL   I. Move right

____ 10. ¶   J. Insert colon

True or False

Mark true statement with a T *and false statements with an* F. *If an answer is "false," rewrite the sentence to make it true.*

____ 1. Modified block, standard, is the most efficient letter style for the ambulatory care setting.

_____

_____

____ 2. Paper for written communications in the office should be of good quality, contain a watermark, and be at least 20-pound stock.

_____

_____

____ 3. A written record of what transpires during a meeting is called the agenda.

_____

_____

____ 4. Business correspondence should be clear, concise, and accurate.

_____

_____

____ 5. First class mail is divided into two mail subclasses.

_____

_____

Processing Mail Exercise

For each type of mail below, list the action the medical assistant should take or to what department or person the medical assistant should forward the mail.

Type of Mail	Action Taken
Invoices for supplies and equipment	_____
Magazines for reception area	_____
Insurance forms	_____
Patient payments	_____
Medical journals	_____
Personal or confidential letters	_____

CERTIFICATION REVIEW

These questions are designed to mimic the certification examination. Select the best response.

1. The "salutation" of a letter is the:

   a. signature

   b. greeting

   c. return address

   d. closing remark (such as: "Sincerely")

   e. the recipient's name, title, and address

2. When addressing an envelope, the proper way to list the state is:

   a. to write it out completely

   b. to abbreviate it using at least the first four letters

   c. to capitalize it using the official two-letter abbreviation

   d. any of the above as long as it is in uppercase letters and is written clearly

3. Which of the below would be incoming mail to a provider's office?

   a. email

   b. insurance forms

   c. medical journals

   d. letters from patients

   e. all of the above

4. The medical assistant may, with the provider's permission, sign certain letters such as:

    a. the ordering of supplies or subscriptions

    b. notification of collection procedures and reminder of payments

    c. dismissal letters

    d. a. and b.

5. When addressing an envelope:

    a. the address should be machine printed with a uniform left margin

    b. all punctuation should be eliminated

    c. use dark ink on a light background using uppercase letters

    d. All of the above

6. The types of envelopes most often used are:

    a. number 7

    b. number 6¾

    c. number 10

    d. b. and c.

7. Periodical is the new term for:

    a. second class mail

    b. third class mail

    c. priority mail

    d. parcel post mail

8. Before presenting any correspondence to the provider for signature, the document should be:

    a. date stamped

    b. checked for accuracy

    c. folded and put in an envelope

    d. typed on plain white paper

9. The most secure service the USPS offers is:

    a. priority mail

    b. express mail

    c. registered mail

    d. certified mail

LEARNING APPLICATION

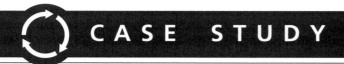

CASE STUDY

Ellen Armstrong, CMA (AAMA), enjoys working on correspondence for Drs. Lewis and King and takes pride in her written communication skills. As an ongoing project, office manager Marilyn Johnson asks Ellen to make suggestions for updating and revising the style manual used in the medical office for written communication guidelines. Ellen suggests the addition of a section in the style manual to discuss bias in language. Bias-free language is sensitive in applying labels to individuals or groups and uses sex-specific words and pronouns appropriately. For example, "dementia" is used instead of "crazy" or "senile." Instead of using "layman," consider using "layperson." Apply "he or she" only in sex-specific usage. Marilyn and the provider-employer ask Ellen to implement the addition to the style manual.

CASE STUDY REVIEW QUESTIONS

1. Why is bias-free language an important consideration in written communication for the ambulatory care setting?

   _____

   _____

   _____

   _____

   _____

2. List other examples of biased language and give suggestions for bias-free alternatives.

   _____

   _____

   _____

   _____

   _____

   _____

Proofreading Exercise

Proofread the letter below, correcting all errors by inserting the proper proofreader's marks directly onto the text. (Consult your textbook for a list of common proofreader's marks and refer to a medical dictionary, if necessary.)

JAMES CARTER, MD, NEUROLOGY
Metropolitan University Medical Center, 8280 Wright Avenue, Northborough, OH 12382

February 2, 20XX

Elizabeth Kind, M.D
Northborough Medical Family Group
The offices of Lewis & King, MD
2501 Center Street
Nrothborough, OH 12345

RE: MARGARET THOMAS

Dear Dr. King:

Thank you for refering Margaret Thomas to my neurological practice. Margaret come to you recently as a new patient for a comprehensive physical examination to evaluate troubling symptoms she had been experiencing for several months. Margaret notices symtoms of tremor, difficulty walking, defective judgement, and hot flushes; she is not able to poinpoint the exac ttime symptoms began. Your physical examination suggested the possible diagnoisis of parkingson's Disease. Margaret presented today for a complete nuerological evaluation.

MEDICAL/SURGICAL HISTORY. The patient is posiitive for the usual childhood diseases and the births of three children, following normal pregnancies. Her surgical history includes an Appendectomy performed 10 years ago. She has a food allergy to shellfish, but no known allergies to medications. She takes Pepto-Bismol and Metamusil for frequent stomach upset and constipation. She is a widow with two children, ages twenty three, twenty-five, and 29, and is a retired homemaker. She does not smoke and has an occassional glass of wine. Her family history is positive for colon cancer in her mother and parenteral grandfather and for lung cancer in her father.

PYHSICALEXAMINATION. VITAL SIGNS: The patient has normal vital signs for a 52-year old Caucasian female. HEENT: The patient had a normacephalic and atraumatic exam. There is mild bobing of the head and facial expressions appear fixed. Pupils equal, round, regular, react to light and acommodation. The fundi were benign. There was normal cup to disc ratio of 0.3. Tympanic Membranes were both clear and mobile. Her nose was clear. the oropharynz ws clear without any evidence of lezions. There was not cervical adenopathy, no thyromegely, or other masses. NECK: Musles of the neck are quite rigid and stiff. CHEST: Cear to percussion and auscultation. HEART: Regular rate and rhythm without murmurs or gallops. there was no jugular venous distention, no peripheral edema, no carotid buits. Pulses were 2+ and symetrical. Abdomen. Some what obese, but benigh. There was not organomegaly or masses. Bowel tones were normal. There was no rebound tenderness. BACK: Examination reveals loss of posturalreflexe and patient stands with head bent forward and wals as if in danger of falling forward. There is difficulty in pivoting and loss of balance. GENITOURINARY: Normal. EXTREMITIES: Thre is moderate bradykinesia. Chracteristic slow, turning motion (pronation-supination) of, the forearm and the hand and a motion of the thumb against the fingers as if rolling a pill between the fingers is noted. This condition seems to worsen when the patient is concentrating or feeling anxious.

continues

(continued)

> **NEUROLOGICAL.** The patient was cooperative and answered all questions. There is no history past of mental disorders or cardiovascular disease. There is muscle weakness and rigidity in all four extremities. Intellect remains intact;
>
> **LABORATORY DATA:** Urinanalysis reveals low levels of dopamin. Cat scan reveals degeneration of nerve cells occuring in the base1 ganglia.
>
> **ASSESSMENT.** Based on the patient history and neurologic examination, it appears most likely that the patient has mild to moderate Parkinsons Disease.
>
> **PLAN.** 1. Recommend physical therapy focussed on learning how to manage diffi- cult movements such as descneding stairs safely.
> 2. Exercises to maintain flexibility, motility, and mental well-being.
> 3. Levadopa to increase dopamine levels in the brain to control symptoms. Please advise the patient that alchohol consumption shoudl be limited because it acts antegonistically to levodopa.
> 4. Relaxation and stress management counseling.
>
> **PROGNOSIS.** Parkinson's disease progresses slowly. Patient should be follow on a regular basis and observed for any signs of damentia which may result in about 1-third of cases.
>
> Sincerely,
>
> James Carter, MD
>
> DD: February 2, 20XX
> DT: February 3, 20XX
> JC/bl

MOSS Activity

Using Medical Office Simulation Software, follow the steps below to generate a letter to a patient. Use the scenario information to compose the body of the letter in full block letter style. When you have finished, print the letter, then fold and insert the letter properly into a correctly addressed envelope.

1. Open MOSS and log in.

2. From the top menu, select Billing, then Patient Ledger.

3. Click on the magnifying glass button next to the Patient Account field.

4. Search for patient Megan Caldwell, and click View.

5. Click on the Correspondence button below the patient ledger.

6. A dialog box will open. Save the file output a location of your choosing which is easily accessible to you, and click OK. Now, a letter template will generate.

7. Compose a letter in full block style, based on the following scenario information. (Hint: Select the text "Type Message Here…." and delete it. Now you are ready to type your letter.)

   • Megan Caldwell's PAP test results were abnormal and Dr. Schwartz would like her to schedule a colposcopy with biopsy in the next few weeks so he can determine the cause of the abnormal results. Please refer to the enclosed brochure for information on this procedure.

8. Proofread the letter for errors, and when you are satisfied that it is complete, save and print the letter.

9. Properly address an envelope to the patient Megan Caldwell.

10. Fold and insert the letter properly into the envelope and turn it in to your instructor.

CHAPTER POST-TEST

Perform this test without looking at your book. If an answer is "false," rewrite the sentence to make it true.

1. The most commonly used of the four major letter styles in the ambulatory care setting is:
   a. full block
   b. modified block, standard
   c. facilitated block, indented
   d. simplified

2. The part of a letter that includes the return address and perhaps a logo is the:
   a. salutation
   b. inside address
   c. letterhead
   d. reference heading
   e. enclosure

3. Whenever documents are to be included in a mailed letter, the word *enclosure* should be indicated by:
   a. Enclosures
   b. Enc.
   c. 1 Enc.
   d. 2 Enclosures
   e. Enclosures (2)
   f. any of the above

4. True or False? Envelopes should be addressed using a combination of uppercase and lowercase letters and with the proper punctuation.

   _____

   _____

5. When it is desirable to send the same letter, although personalized, to many different people, a computerized feature that can be used is called:
   a. word processing letters
   b. mail merge
   c. database letters
   d. merge correspondence

6. True or False? Only the first letter of the first word in the complimentary closing is uppercase.

   _____

   _____

SELF-ASSESSMENT

In your written communications, are you able to express yourself accurately and concisely? Able to communicate ideas effectively? Capable of proofreading and editing for content? Use this simple self-assessment to gauge your comfort and proficiency in written communications by identifying strengths and pinpointing any weak areas that could use improvement. For each statement below, circle the corresponding letter to the response that best describes you.

1. When writing a letter, I generally feel:

   a. confident. I communicate effectively on the page and enjoy writing letters.

   b. at ease. My written communication skills are acceptable.

   c. uncomfortable. I would rather communicate verbally than through writing.

2. As far as content goes, when I am given the required information and asked to compose a letter, I:

   a. almost always understand exactly what I am being asked to communicate and am able to convey it precisely in letter form

   b. generally understand what I am being asked to communicate, but sometimes have to fine-tune my letters

   c. often have trouble understanding what I am being asked to communicate and usually have to go back and ask questions about the letter's content

3. In general, when choosing words for written correspondence, I feel:

   a. secure about my ability to select appropriate language and use medical terminology accurately

   b. pretty confident, although my general vocabulary and knowledge of medical terminology could use some improvement

   c. frustrated; I always seem to confuse words and medical terms no matter how hard I try not to

4. As far as spelling goes, I am:

   a. a top-notch speller; I always keep both a standard and medical dictionary on hand for the words I am not sure of

   b. an adequate speller; sometimes I confuse a word here or there; I always have to proofread carefully for spelling errors

   c. a below-par speller; my letters are always littered with misspellings and someone else has to proofread my work

5. Grammatically speaking, I am:

   a. above average; I routinely find mistakes in my colleagues' work

   b. passable; I make minor mistakes but usually catch them while proofreading

   c. hopeless; people find mistakes in my work even after I have checked it twice

6. Regarding proofreader's marks, I am:

   a. highly capable of proofreading my work; if colleagues need someone to proof their work, I am first on their list

   b. an okay proofreader; I occasionally overlook a mistake, but nobody's perfect

   c. frightened; proofreading marks are just a bunch of meaningless squiggles to me

7. How would you describe your formatting skills?

    a. Exemplary. I understand all basic letter forms, and all of my letters are rigorously formatted according to correct specifications.

    b. Satisfactory. Every so often, I confuse styles or forget an annotation; but in general, all my letters are formatted correctly.

    c. Fair to nonexistent. I have trouble understanding why every letter has to be so formally constructed.

8. When adhering to office style guidelines, I:

    a. always follow the guidelines

    b. usually have no problem sticking to style guidelines; when I make a mistake, it is a rare event

    c. need improvement; my letters are frequently littered with style inconsistencies, and I do not understand the need for an office style as long as each letter is written with accurate information

9. Overall, I think of writing letters in the health care environment as:

    a. one of my strong suits

    b. a task that I am able to accomplish, just not one I particularly enjoy

    c. a necessary evil

Scoring: If your answers were mostly A responses, you have strong written communications skills and enjoy writing letters. If your responses were mostly Bs, your written communications skills are good but could stand some improvement. Try reviewing pertinent information in this chapter to strengthen areas that need it. If your answers were mostly Cs, you need to work on your written communication skills. Volunteer to take on as many written correspondence assignments as you can—practice may help you overcome your apprehension about writing letters and will almost certainly raise the quality of your work.

_____

_____

_____

_____

_____

_____

_____

_____

_____

C H A P T E R **16**

Medical Documents

CHAPTER PRE-TEST

Perform this test without looking at your book. If an answer is "false," rewrite the sentence to make it true.

1. True or False? Outsourcing is rapidly eliminating the need for the traditional transcriptionists in medical facilities.

   _____

   _____

2. True or False? Anyone who has computer abilities and can spell well can perform medical transcription well.

   _____

   _____

3. True or False? Medical documents are only for the clinic and provider who generated them, so they are called "internal documents."

   _____

   _____

4. True or False? Medical transcription is a profession that has not really undergone many changes in the last decade or so.

   _____

   _____

5. True or False? If a medical transcriptionist encounters a term that cannot be interpreted or something new that cannot be referenced, that section of the document should be flagged.

   _____

   _____

6. True or False? Medical transcriptionists do not need to be concerned with HIPAA regulations.

   _____

   _____

VOCABULARY BUILDER

Find the words below that are misspelled; circle them, and correctly spell them in the spaces provided. Then insert the correct vocabulary terms from the list that best fit the descriptions below.

athentication	discharge summery	priveliged
autapsy report	editor	progress notes
chart notes	electronic health records	proofreading
chief complaint	gross examination	quality assurance
confidentility	history and physical	review of symptoms
consultation reports	medical transcriptionist	risk management
correspondence	outsourcing	turnaround time
currant	patholigy	voice recognition software

_____   _____   _____

_____   _____   _____

_____   _____   _____

1. Today, the _____ may be more involved with quality assurance than actually transcribing medical records, notes, letters, and documents.

2. The part of the pathology report that describes the size and shape of a biopsy is called a _____.

3. The part of patients' hospital records that describe their entire hospital stay, progress, and condition on release is called a _____.

4. The part of the patient's medical record that contains information related to the main reason for the encounter, as well as a synopsis of the patient's previous medical information, is called the _____.

5. Reports such as history and physicals that should be completed within 24 hours are called _____ reports.

6. A type of signature that may use various computer key entries as identification is referred to as _____.

7. Software that translates spoken sounds into written words is called _____.

8. A medical report generated to describe the examinations of tissues or cells obtained through a surgery or medical procedure is the _____ report.

9. The practice of contracting transcription with a service outside of the clinic or hospital to a company where it can be done at a lower cost and with a faster turnaround time is called _____.

Definitions

Define the following terms.

1. Joint Commission:

_____

_____

_____

2. Consultation report:

_____

_____

_____

_____

3. Editing:

_____

_____

4. Flag:

_____

_____

_____

5. Turnaround time:

_____

_____

_____

_____

LEARNING REVIEW

Short Answer

1. List five personal attributes of the medical transcriptionist.

_____

_____

_____

_____

_____

2. Give two examples of each type of turnaround time report and the time of the turnaround.

STAT _____   _____

Current _____   _____

Old _____   _____

3. List at least four advantages of outsourcing.

_____

_____

_____

_____

_____

4. Offices using electronic medical records may delegate much of the medical transcriptionist's responsibility to other medical personnel. Identify the items below that may be entered into an electronic medical record by the medical assistant by writing (MA) next to the entry, and those items that may be entered by the provider (P).

Reason for the patient's visit _____

Entering chart notes _____

Entering vital signs _____

Entering and transmitting prescription to a pharmacy _____

Transmitting the medical record to another provider _____

Entering current medications _____

Entering the chief complaint _____

Abbreviations Exercise

Write what each abbreviation stands for.

1. EHR _____

2. MT _____

3. TAT _____

4. QA _____

5. VRS _____

6. CMT _____

7. CC _____

8. ROS _____

9. H&P _____

10. DS _____

11. OR _____

12. HIPAA _____

True or False

Mark a true statement with a T *and a false statement with an* F. *If an answer is "false," rewrite the sentence to make it true.*

____ 1. Medical records are documents governed by laws and may be subpoenaed for review by various courts.

_____

_____

____ 2. The medical report may play a major role in substantiating injury or a malpractice claim.

_____

_____

____ 3. The Joint Commission allows 36 hours from admission for a history and physical report to be dictated, transcribed, and filed into the patient's medical record.

_____

_____

____ 4. When transcribing radiology or imaging reports, the date of service should be used rather than the date of dictation.

_____

_____

____ 5. Electronic signatures on medical documents are allowed by both Medicare and the Joint Commission.

_____

_____

____ 6. When editing the transcribed document, it may be necessary to change the dictator's style or meaning.

_____

_____

____ 7. Once a job has been accepted, the transcriptionist or transcription service is legally bound to meet the schedule, short of "an act of nature."

_____

_____

____ 8. Meeting deadlines is irrelevant and there is not stringent adherence to turnaround time.

_____

_____

____ 9. Risk management personnel should be consulted first before divulging files to an attorney or insurance representative.

_____

_____

____ 10. Provider-directors or office managers should not be responsible for the wrongful acts of medical transcriptionists working under their supervision.

_____

_____

CERTIFICATION REVIEW

These questions are designed to mimic the certification examination. Select the best response.

1. Association for Healthcare Documentation Integrity (AHDI) credentials _____.

   a. MTs

   b. CMTs

   c. CMTs and RMTs

   d. CMAs and RMAs

2. A digital dictation system allows you to measure to:

   a. the 30th or 90th of a minute

   b. 60 seconds

   c. the 10th or 100th of a minute

   d. 30–40 seconds

3. The medical report must be:

   a. dated correctly

   b. signed or initialed by the dictator

   c. legible

   d. all of the above

4. The specific time period in which a document is expected to be completed from the time it is received by the transcriptionist until it is returned to the provider and made part of the permanent medical record is called:

   a. filing time

   b. turnaround time

   c. completion time

   d. return time

5. Radiology, pathology, and laboratory reports are usually termed as _____ to indicate the need for immediate turnaround.

   a. ASAP

   b. current

   c. old

   d. STAT

LEARNING APPLICATION

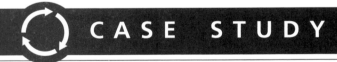

CASE STUDY

You are transcribing a report when you notice it is a report about your neighbor. The report states that the test run for multiple sclerosis is positive. You had just spoken to your neighbor yesterday and she was concerned that she hadn't heard from her provider and was wondering about the results of her tests.

CASE STUDY REVIEW QUESTIONS

1. What should you do?

   _____

   _____

   _____

   _____

   _____

Proofreading Exercise

Correct the following paragraph.

```
her past medical history is postivie for the usual childhood diseases and the births of to
children following normal pregnancies she has a negative pasts urgical history. she has
no allergies To medications and takes tylenol for occasional headashes She is married
and has to children, ages 3 and 12 months. She does not smoke or drink
```

CHAPTER POST-TEST

Perform this test without looking at your book. If an answer is "false," rewrite the sentence to make it true.

1. True or False? The need for the traditional medical transcriptionist in a medical facility today is declining due to outsourcing.

   _____

   _____

2. True or False? Medical transcription is a job for people with good computer abilities and word processing speed; who have excellent spelling, grammar, and punctuation skills; and who care enough to do the best job possible.

   _____

   _____

3. True or False? Medical documents are not only for the clinic and provider who generated them, they are also legal documents used by many professionals.

   _____

   _____

4. True or False? Medical transcription is a profession that has undergone numerous changes in the last decade or so.

   _____

   _____

5. True or False? If a medical transcriptionist cannot interpret a portion of the sentence or cannot make reference, then that portion of the document should be flagged.

   _____

   _____

6. True or False? Because medical transcriptionists work within the medical field with medical information, they need to be concerned with HIPAA regulations.

   _____

   _____

SELF-ASSESSMENT

1. Do you think you would enjoy working as a transcriptionist? What is it about the profession that appeals to you? What is it about the profession that does not appeal to you?

_____

_____

_____

_____

_____

C H A P T E R **17**

Medical Insurance

CHAPTER PRE-TEST

Perform this test without looking at your book. If an answer is "false," rewrite the sentence to make it true.

1. True or False? Managed care has simplified the patient's responsibility for payment.

_____

_____

2. True or False? With managed care options, there is less emphasis on the medical assistant needing to be accurate and timely when filing insurance claims.

_____

_____

3. True or False? Preexisting conditions usually require a waiting period.

_____

_____

4. True or False? "Coordination of benefits" means that the insurance companies will take care of the paperwork.

_____

_____

5. True or False? Co-payment is the amount the insurance will cost the patient each month.

_____

_____

VOCABULARY BUILDER

Misspelled Words

Find the words below that are misspelled; circle them, and correctly spell them in the spaces provided. Then, insert the correct vocabulary terms from the list that best fit the descriptions below.

ajustment

preautherization

referral

benefit period

prefered provider organization

resourse-based relative value scale

Medicare Part D

primary care provider

self-insurance

point-of-service plan

proof of eligability

usual, customarry, and reasonable

_____   _____   _____

_____   _____   _____

1. The _____ is a doctor chosen by the patient who is the first doctor the patient sees and is responsible for making referrals for further treatment by a specialist or for hospitalization.

2. A _____ allows the enrollee to have the freedom to obtain medical care from an HMO provider or to self-refer to a non-HMO provider at a greater cost.

3. The _____ was developed using values for each medical and surgical procedure based on work, practice, and malpractice costs and factoring in the regional differences.

4. _____ means that prior notice and approval needs to be obtained before services will be covered.

5. A _____ is an organization of providers who network together to offer discounts to purchasers of health care insurance.

6. The _____ is the specified time during which benefits will be paid under certain types of health insurance coverages.

7. The amount a provider writes off the patient's account is known as an _____.

8. _____ is prescription drug coverage by Medicare.

Abbreviations Exercise

List what each of the following acronyms stands for.

1. CMS _____

2. COB _____

3. DEERS _____

4. EPO _____

5. HMO _____

6. IDS _____

7. MCO _____

8. POS _____

9. PPO _____

10. UCR _____

LEARNING REVIEW

Short Answer

1. What questions should the medical assistant ask when screening for medical insurance coverage?

_____

_____

_____

2. What measures do managed care organizations employ to ensure cost-effective services?

_____

_____

_____

3. What are the six models of managed care organizations in use?

_____

_____

_____

4. List seven pieces of information that should be maintained in a log regarding preauthorization, precertification, or referral procedures for various insurance carriers.

_____

_____

_____

_____

_____

5. Identify the three common elements involved in computing a provider's fee schedule.

_____

_____

_____

6. The insurance carrier generates an EOB and an RA. Explain what these are and who they are sent to.

_____

_____

_____

_____

_____

7. List three examples of insurance fraud, and three examples of insurance abuse.

A. Fraud:

_____

_____

_____

_____

B: Abuse:

_____

_____

_____

_____

Matching

Match the statements below to the appropriate Medicare Part.

_____ 1. Covers outpatient expenses including providers' fees, lab tests, and radiologic studies

_____ 2. Covers hospital admission and stays

_____ 3. Offers prescription drug coverage for everyone covered by Medicare

_____ 4. Referred to as Medicare advantage plans

_____ 5. Does not require a monthly premium

_____ 6. Has a "donut hole" or coverage gap

_____ 7. Will start paying for services after a $131 deductible has been met

_____ 8. Requires a monthly premium

_____ 9. Covers hospice care

_____ 10. Covers charges for durable medical equipment

A. Medicare Part A

B. Medicare Part B

C. Medicare Part C

D. Medicare Part D

CERTIFICATION REVIEW

These questions are designed to mimic the certification examination. Select the best response.

1. The portion of the medical fees that the patient needs to pay at the time of services is called:

a. co-pay

b. fee for service

c. out-of-pocket expenses

d. premium

2. The largest medical insurance program in the United States is:

   a. Blue Cross/Blue Shield

   b. Medicaid

   c. Medicare

   d. TRICARE

3. The cost that patients must pay each month (sometimes provided by their employers) is called the:

   a. out-of-pocket expense

   b. co-pay

   c. premium

   d. relative value scale

4. Which of the following describes HIPAA?

   a. It is about confidentiality, patient privacy, and security of personal health information.

   b. It protects health insurance coverage for workers and their families when they change or lose their jobs.

   c. It includes national standards for electronic health care transactions.

   d. It establishes rules for national identifiers for providers, health plans, and employers.

   e. a. and c. only

5. Noncovered services are also known as:

   a. nonallowed services

   b. exclusions

   c. out-of-pocket services

   d. expensive services

6. A statement summarizing how the insurance carrier determined reimbursement for services received by the patient is called a(n):

   a. EOB

   b. RA

   c. day sheet

   d. personal financial statement

7. The medical insurance that covers medical care for certain qualifying low-income individuals is:

   a. Medicare

   b. CHAMPUS

   c. TRICARE

   d. Medicaid

8. To ensure that there is a successful flow of adequate income in the clinic or office, the medical assistant should:

   a. bill the insurance carrier or patient as needed

   b. complete forms properly

   c. keep track of aging accounts

   d. All of the above

9. Improper billing practices are considered:

   a. fraud

   b. nonproductive

   c. abuse

   d. risky

10. Which of the following is a problem with work-related health insurance coverage?

    a. Part-time employees are usually not eligible.

    b. Medical benefits may not transfer equally.

    c. Insurance companies often refuse to provide coverage for some procedures, including experimental treatments.

    d. All of the above

11. The person covered under the terms of an insurance policy is called the:

    a. primary

    b. secondary

    c. beneficiary

    d. elector

12. When more than one policy covers the individual, the _____ determines which of the policies will pay first.

    a. deductible

    b. exclusion

    c. coinsurance

    d. coordination of benefits

13. Where does one find the address to which insurance claims are to be sent?

    a. The telephone book

    b. On the back of the insurance card

    c. In the insurance provider manual

    d. None of the above

14. Blue Cross and Blue Shield are examples of:

    a. MCOs

    b. HMOs

    c. PPOs

    d. traditional insurance organizations

LEARNING APPLICATION

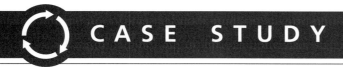

CASE STUDY

Lourdes Austen, a one-year survivor of breast cancer, is covered by an HMO. Lourdes's primary care provider, Dr. King, recommends that Lourdes receive a colonoscopy because she has a family history that is positive for colon cancer, and medical studies have demonstrated a link between colon and breast cancers in families. Lourdes's HMO requires preauthorization before a specialist's care can be provided. Dr. King supplies the referral to a gastroenterologist who will perform the colon screening test and gives Lourdes the necessary completed referral form to take with her to her scheduled appointment. During the colonoscopy procedure, one benign polyp is removed, and the gastroenterologist requests that Lourdes return for a follow-up examination in one week.

Lourdes makes an appointment with the specialist's administrative medical assistant. When she returns one week later, the medical assistant informs Lourdes that she must have a new referral form for the office visit or the HMO will not approve payment; Lourdes will have to pay for the examination herself. "But we drove 40 minutes to get here, and no one ever told me I'd need another form for this. I thought it was all covered under the colonoscopy," Lourdes says.

CASE STUDY REVIEW QUESTIONS

1. Lourdes's HMO policy requires preauthorization. Is there anything that can be done to secure a proper referral without having to schedule another appointment for the patient or force the patient to pay for the office visit?

_____

_____

_____

_____

_____

2. What is the role of the specialist's administrative medical assistant in this situation? Could the situation have been prevented?

_____

_____

_____

_____

_____

CHAPTER POST-TEST

Perform this test without looking at your book. If an answer is "false," rewrite the sentence to make it true.

1. True or False? Managed care has made the patient's responsibility for payment more complex.

   _____

   _____

2. True or False? With managed care options, there is more emphasis on the medical assistant needing to be accurate and timely when filing insurance claims.

   _____

   _____

3. True or False? Preexisting conditions always require a waiting period.

   _____

   _____

4. True or False? "Coordination of benefits" means that the insurance companies will handle all the paperwork necessary for payment.

   _____

   _____

5. True or False? Co-payment is the amount the insurance will cost the patient's employer each month.

   _____

   _____

SELF-ASSESSMENT

1. Take a close look at your insurance coverage. If you do not have medical insurance coverage, take a look at the coverage of a close friend or relative or choose a policy you would like to have.

   A. Does it require a co-pay?

   B. How much is the co-pay for a doctor's visit?

   C. How much is the co-pay or a hospital stay? surgery?

   D. How much is the co-pay for medication?

   E. Does prescribed medication have to be from a formulary list?

   F. How much is the total amount you would have to pay for any given year?

2. Some people advocate doing away with health insurance for office visits and medications and just having insurance for big expenses such as catastrophic coverage. Discuss this idea with a group of at least three people. These people may be your classmates or friends/family. Write up a list of the advantages and disadvantages.

   _____

   _____

   _____

   _____

3. Some people advocate a "socialistic" method of health insurance such as Canada has. Look online for information about Canada's health care system and make a list of the advantages and disadvantages. Which way would you vote if you had a choice?

_____

_____

_____

_____

CHAPTER **19**

Daily Financial Practices

CHAPTER PRE-TEST

Perform this test without looking at your book. If an answer is "false," rewrite the sentence to make it true.

1. True or False? The management of the business details of a practice usually becomes the responsibility of the medical assisting staff.

   _____

   _____

2. True or False? Every patient, regardless of insurance coverage, should be charged the same fee for the same service.

   _____

   _____

3. True or False? You should discourage the use of credit/debit cards for making payments for services rendered.

   _____

   _____

4. True or False? Purchase orders are to be written up when the purchase arrives.

   _____

   _____

5. True or False? Petty cash is available for authorized use when the purchase is minor or unexpected and when a check is not necessary.

   _____

   _____

VOCABULARY BUILDER

Misspelled Words

Find the words below that are misspelled; circle them, and correctly spell them in the spaces provided. Then insert correct vocabulary terms from the list that best fit into the descriptive sentence below.

accounts payible	debit	payee
accounts recievable	dispursements	pegboard system
adjustments	encounter form	petty cash
balance	guaranter	posting
cashier's check	leadger	traveler's check
certified check	money market account	voucher check
credit	National Provider Identifier	
day sheet	notary	

_____   _____   _____

_____   _____

_____ 1. A record of daily patient transactions used in conjunction with pegboard systems

_____ 2. Small cash sum kept on hand in the office for minor or unexpected expenses

_____ 3. Decreases the balance due

_____ 4. Replaces all other identifiers used by providers for reimbursement and other transactions with private payers and the government

_____ 5. As a noun, this term denotes "the amount owed"; as a verb, the term means "to verify posting accuracy"

_____ 6. Accounting function that describes the act of recording financial transactions into bookkeeping or accounting systems

_____ 7. Increases or decreases to a patient account not due to charges incurred or payments received

_____ 8. Sum owed by a business for services or goods received

_____ 9. Sum owed to a business for services or goods supplied

LEARNING REVIEW

Short Answer

1. Identify two work guidelines essential to creating and maintaining accurate financial records.

_____

_____

2. Identify six habits essential to creating and maintaining accurate paper financial records.

_____

_____

_____

_____

_____

3. Identify seven of the nine features that may be a part of the checking account.

_____

_____

_____

_____

_____

4. What are five rules to ensure that checks are properly written and recorded?

_____

_____

_____

_____

_____

5. Give three reasons why it is important to ensure that proper control is utilized when purchasing supplies and equipment.

_____

_____

_____

6. When office supplies arrive, what should be done to verify that the correct items and quantities have been received? What should be done to prepare the invoice for payment?

_____

_____

_____

_____

_____

_____

_____

7. Describe the following types of checks, which are different from checks issued from a standard business checking account.

    (1) Cashier's check:

    _____

    _____

    _____

    (2) Certified check:

    _____

    _____

    _____

    (3) Money order:

    _____

    _____

    _____

    (4) Voucher check:

    _____

    _____

    _____

    _____

    (5) Traveler's check:

    _____

    _____

8. Adjustments are entries made to a patient's account that do not represent charges or payments. Name three reasons why adjustments may sometimes be made to a patient's account.

    _____

    _____

    _____

9. Deposits are generally made daily. All checks to be deposited must be endorsed. Define endorsement. Identify the best method of endorsing checks in the ambulatory care setting and describe the benefits of using this method.

    _____

    _____

    _____

    _____

    _____

10. Checks received from patients and others must be inspected before preparing the checks for deposit. What guidelines should medical assistants follow in accepting and inspecting checks?

    _____

    _____

    _____

11. If a check is returned to the ambulatory care setting for insufficient funds, what procedures should be followed?

_____

_____

_____

12. It is crucial to balance all financial information for each day and for the month's end. Month-end figures on the day sheet must agree with the patient ledgers. Why is it important to go through this time-consuming accounting process?

_____

_____

_____

_____

_____

_____

_____

CERTIFICATION REVIEW

These questions are designed to mimic the certification examination. Select the best response.

1. The pegboard system of bookkeeping is sometimes called the:

   a. write-it-once system

   b. ledger system

   c. double-entry system

   d. duplicated page system

2. NSF stands for:

   a. nonsufficient funds

   b. not sufficient funds

   c. not satisfactory funding

   d. negligent status of funding

3. A restrictive endorsement stamp is used to:

   a. stamp on the ledger to signify that payment has been made

   b. stamp the doctor's signature on insurance forms and other documents

   c. stamp on the statement to signify that you have sent a check

   d. stamp on the back of a check to signify "for deposit only"

4. When reconciling a bank statement:

   a. the reconciling should be done every month

   b. the checkbook entries should be checked against the bank statement

   c. the reconciling should be done daily by computer

   d. all reconciling should be done in ink to avoid any unauthorized entries

   e. a. and b.

5. If a check has been deposited and is now returned due to insufficient funds, it will be necessary to:

   a. redeposit the check

   b. call the bank that returned it and verify availability of funds so the check can then be redeposited

   c. call the patient who wrote the check

   d. discard the check and credit the amount back to the patient's account

6. The most common method(s) of tracking a patient's balance is (are):

   a. the pegboard system

   b. computerized financial systems

   c. the ledger card

   d. a. and b.

7. The pegboard system consists of:

   a. day sheets

   b. ledger cards

   c. encounter forms

   d. receipt forms

   e. All of the above

8. In cases of divorced parents where one parent has physical custody of the child and is considered the one responsible for payment if the child is not insured with a contracted insurance carrier, the parent is called:

   a. the payee

   b. the guarantor

   c. the subscriber

   d. none of the above

9. The number required by the Centers for Medicare & Medicaid Services (CMS) on claims for clinical diagnosis services is called the:

   a. insurance registration number

   b. client number

   c. National Provider Identifier

   d. contract number

10. The Advanced Beneficiary Notification form is used primarily for:

    a. Medicaid patients

    b. HMO patients

    c. Medicare patients for the purpose of collecting payments that are not allowed

    d. CHAMPUS patients

11. A patient encounter form:

    a. is also called a charge slip

    b. is also called a superbill

    c. is also called a pegboard form

    d. both a. and b.

12. In most practices there is a need to have cash available on a daily basis to:

    a. make change for a patient paying cash for services

    b. make funds available for all office personnel

    c. pay for minor and incidental expenses

    d. provide funds for weekly lunches for all employees

13. When a check must be guaranteed for the amount in which it is written, a _____ is issued.

    a. cashier's check

    b. certified check

    c. voucher check

    d. traveler's check

14. Restricting the use of a check should it be lost or stolen may be done through:

    a. reconciling

    b. balancing

    c. special endorsement

    d. blank endorsement

LEARNING APPLICATION

Hands-on Activities

1. Administrative medical assistant Karen Ritter is responsible for assisting the office manager and accountant in performing accounts payable activities for Inner City Health Care. On September 4, she receives a $323.45 bill from RJ Medical Supply Company for blood pressure equipment the office received on August 30. Noting that the company demands payment within 30 days of billing, Karen writes a check disbursing funds to the company on September 15. The balance in the office's checking account before this check is written is $26,100.00. Using this information, write out the check and stub below. Karen will submit the check to Susan Rice, M.D., for her signature.

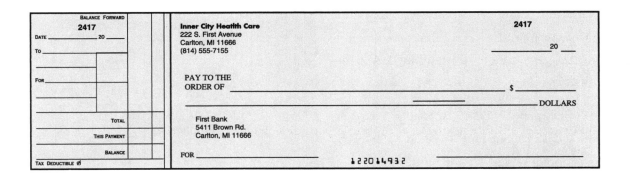

2. Office manager Walter Seals, CMA (AAMA), is responsible for purchasing office supplies for Inner City Health Care. On September 10, Walter completes purchase order #1742 to Mayflower Supply, requested by administrative medical assistant Karen Ritter. The items are taxed at 8%, and the shipping fee is prepaid. The items are billed and shipped to Inner City Health Care; the terms are net due 30 days. Complete the purchase order form below.

PURCHASE ORDER

NO. 1742

Bill To:	Ship To:	Vendor:

REQ BY	BUYER	TERMS

QTY	ITEM	UNITS	DESCRIPTION	UNIT PR	TOTAL
					SUBTOTAL
					TAX
					FREIGHT
					BAL DUE

Inner City Health Care   Mayflower Supply, Inc.

222 S. First Avenue   642 East 65th Street

Carlton, MI 11666   Carlton, MI 11623

(814) 555-7155   (814) 555-9999

2 boxes of fax paper, #62145, at $8.99 a box

5 day-view desk calendars, #24598, at $4.25 each

4 cases of copier paper, #72148, at $20.00 a case

5 boxes of highlighter pens, 12 to a box, #26773, at $3.98 a box

4 computer printer cartridges, #96187, at $49.99 each

MOSS Activities

1. Using Medical Office Simulation Software and the skills learned in Procedure 19-3, post procedure charges for the following patients. If a patient has a co-payment due, post the co-payment at the time of procedure posting.

A. Edward Gormann was seen in the office on July 10, 2009, complaining of an earache.

Reference Number	1010
Office Visit Type	Established patient, expanded problem-focused (99213)
Diagnosis Codes	Otitis media (382.9)
Co-payment	The patient pays his $20.00 with a check, #751, at the time of service.

B. Julia Martin was seen in the office on July 10, 2009, complaining of heartburn.

Reference Number	1011
Office Visit Type	New patient, problem-focused (99203)
Diagnosis Codes	Gastroesophageal reflux (530.81)

C. Megan Caldwell was seen in the office on July 15, 2009 to check for strep throat.

Reference Number	1035
Office Visit Type	Established patient, problem-focused (99212)
Procedures	Rapid strep test (87880)
Diagnosis	Strep throat (034.0)
Co-payment	The patient pays her $20.00 with cash at the time of service.

D. Remi Beaufort was seen in the office on July 15, 2009 for a mono screen.

Reference Number	1036
Office Visit Type	New patient, expanded problem focused (99202)
Procedure Codes	Mono screen (86308)
Diagnosis Codes	Mononucleosis (075)
Co-payment	The patient's father pays the $20.00 with a check, #1056, at the time of service.

2. Using Medical Office Simulation Software and the skills learned in Procedure 19-4, perform insurance billing for the procedures posted in the first exercise, for patients Gormann, Martin, Caldwell, and Beaufort.

A. Choose Electronic for the Transmit Type.

B. Print or save the prebilling worksheet for each patient to be turned in to your instructor.

C. Print or save the resulting transmission report to be turned in to your instructor.

3. Using Medical Office Simulation Software and the skills learned in Procedure 19-5, post insurance payments for the same group of payments.

   A. The office receives an EOB from Flexihealth PPO InNetwork on July 30, 2009:

      • For patient Edward Gormann, the plan allowable was $98.24 less the patient's $20 co-pay. The net amount the plan paid for the visit was $78.24 (post an insurance adjustment of $12.76).
      • For patient Megan Caldwell, for the 99212 charge, the plan allowable was $70.80 less the patient's $20 co-pay. The net amount the plan paid for this charge was $50.80 (post an insurance adjustment of $9.20). For the rapid strep test, the plan allowable was $40.71 (post an insurance adjustment of $5.29).

   B. The office receives an EOB from ConsumerOne HRA on July 24, 2009, for Julia Martin's charge. The plan allowable was $177. Write off the remaining amount as an insurance adjustment.

   C. The office receives a RA from Signal HRA on July 31, 2009, for Remi Beaufort's charges. For the 99202 charge, the plan allowable was $130, less the patient's $10 co-pay. The net amount the plan paid for this charge was $110 (post an insurance adjustment of $27). For the mono screen, the plan allowable was $15.05 (post an insurance adjustment of $1.95).

CHAPTER POST-TEST

Perform this test without looking at your book. If an answer is "false," rewrite the sentence to make it true.

1. True or False? The management of the business details of a practice usually becomes the responsibility of the medical assisting staff.

2. True or False? The same fees for services should be charged to every patient, regardless of whether they have insurance coverage.

3. True or False? You should encourage the use of credit/debit cards for medical bills.

4. True or False? Purchase orders are to be written up before the purchase is made.

5. True or False? Petty cash is available for authorized use when employees need cash for minor, routine, or small unexpected expenses.

SELF-ASSESSMENT

1. In your personal checkbook or banking system at home, how often do you reconcile?

_____

_____

_____

_____

2. When you do reconcile, do you balance? How much time will you spend on the reconciliation to balance? If you reconcile your bank statements on a regular basis and balance each month, congratulations! If you do not reconcile on a regular basis, start today. Gather your last bank statement. If you do not have one, call the bank and have them send you one or download one from the Internet if your bank offers Internet banking. Accept the beginning balance on the bank statement. Gather the check stubs/copies that you have written within the bank statement's beginning and end dates. Check off all the checks that have gone through the bank and are listed on the statement.

   Add up the outstanding checks (i.e., the ones that have not gone through yet). Subtract them from the ending balance. Add in any interest you have earned for the month. Subtract any fees you have been charged. Does your amount match the bank statement? If not, go back over your math to make sure you added and subtracted correctly and fix any errors. If you still cannot balance, call the bank and ask to sit down with a representative/clerk so they can help you balance. After you balance once, the next month will be much easier. If your bank offers Internet or online banking, and you are not using that option, consider it. Why are you not using it? Talk to a representative to be sure the online service is secure and your information is protected. If you are satisfied that it is a safe and secure service, consider taking advantage of the online option. Reconciling the monthly statements online is easy to do because the math is done for you by the computer! If you are using online banking, do you think it saves you time? Does it save you money? Is it easier than reconciling manually?

_____

_____

_____

_____

_____

C H A P T E R **2 0**

Billing and Collections

CHAPTER PRE-TEST

Perform this test without looking at your book. If an answer is "false," rewrite the sentence to make it true.

1. The Truth-in-Lending Act states:

   a. Providers cannot charge more than 10% interest on their patient accounts.

   b. Providers must charge interest if the account is more than four months past due.

   c. Providers must notify patients in writing if interest is to be charged on their accounts.

   d. If the provider and patient agree to an installment plan of more than four payments, the installment charge must be stated in writing.

2. True or False? The best opportunity for collection is at the time of services.

   _____

   _____

3. True or False? Large clinics with numerous statements to send out each month will find the monthly billing cycle method to be the most efficient.

   _____

   _____

4. True or False? A collection ratio of 80% is considered a good ratio.

   _____

   _____

VOCABULARY BUILDER

Misspelled Words

Find the words below that are misspelled; circle them, and correctly spell them in the spaces provided. Then match the correct vocabulary term to its definition below.

accounts recievable ratio   collection ratio   statute of limatations

collection agency   probate court   Truth-in-Lending Act

_____   _____

_____   1. Also known as the Consumer Protection Act of 1967; an act requiring providers of installment credits to state the charges in writing and to express the interest as an annual rate

_____   2. An outside establishment that collects outstanding debt

_____   3. Defines the period of time in which legal action can take place

_____   4. Shows the status of collections and the possible losses in a medical facility

_____   5. A measure of how effective collections are and an indication of how quickly outstanding accounts are paid

LEARNING REVIEW

Short Answer

1. A billing efficiency report allows for careful monitoring of follow-up bills; that is, whether they were paid, if the insurance has paid, and an assessment of the patient's responsibility for payment. What five pieces of data are included in these reports from which production efficiency is calculated?

_____

_____

_____

2. Identify and explain the five most common reasons some patient accounts become past due.

_____

_____

_____

_____

_____

_____

3. In the pegboard system, what method is used to identify the age of accounts?

_____

_____

_____

_____

_____

4. Name five criteria according to which computer programs can age accounts.

_____

_____

_____

5. The computer can also generate accounts receivable reports. Name three pieces of information included on a computer-generated accounts receivable report.

_____

_____

6. Collection agencies generally provide two services to an ambulatory care facility. Name and describe each type of service.

_____

_____

_____

_____

_____

7. Collection of fees when a patient has died is directed to the executor of the estate. Place an X next to each action below that represents a responsible action in collecting past due accounts from deceased patients' estates.

_____ If there is no known administrator, address the statement to "Estate of [insert patient's name]" and mail to the patient's last known address.

_____ Send an invoice via certified mail with a complete breakdown of all monies owed by the deceased patient's spouse or closest relative, noting that the survivor is responsible for making payment in full.

_____ Mail the account information via certified mail, return receipt, to the administrator of the estate, whose name can be obtained from the probate department of superior court.

_____ If unsure how to proceed, contact the office's attorney or the probate court for advice.

8. With regard to collections, the statute of limitations is usually defined by the class of the overdue account. Name the three classes of accounts.

_____

_____

_____

9. There are certain legal rules and ethical guidelines to follow when placing collection calls. Circle all that apply.

(1) Callers must identify themselves and validate that the person they are talking to is the responsible party.

(2) Threaten to turn the call over to a collection agency.

(3) Do not call the patient's place of employment.

(4) Do not make repeated calls to the debtor's friends or family.

True or False?

Mark a true statement with a T *and a false statement with an* F. *If an answer is "false," rewrite the sentence to make it true.*

____ 1. Most states regulate the time frame when collection calls can be placed, which is usually between the hours of 8 AM and 8 PM.

_____

_____

____ 2. Emancipated minors are responsible for their own accounts.

_____

_____

____ 3. The expense of hiring an outside collection agency may not always justify the amount of fees to be collected.

_____

_____

____ 4. Not all accounts can be collected, so it is best to identify them early, write them off, and save the practice time and money.

_____

_____

____ 5. An account assigned to a collection agency can be filed in small claims court.

_____

_____

CERTIFICATION REVIEW

These questions are designed to mimic the certification examination. Select the best response.

1. Patients who owe money but have moved and left no forwarding address are referred to as:

   a. deadbeats

   b. skips

   c. nonpayers

   d. dead accounts

2. Statutes of limitations vary from state to state but should be investigated if an unpaid account is more than:

   a. 3 years old

   b. 5 years old

   c. 10 years old

   d. without a time limit if the account is more than a certain amount

3. Lack of payment from a patient may not be considered serious until after:

   a. 30 days

   b. 60 days

   c. 90 days

   d. 120 days

4. For an insurance claim pending more than 45 days, the medical assistant should:

   a. call the carrier and find out if the claim was received

   b. rebill the insurance company

   c. check on the processing status of the claim with the carrier

   d. a. and c.

5. The most appropriate time to discuss fees for financial concerns of the patient is:

   a. when services are rendered

   b. when scheduling an appointment

   c. by mail after services are rendered

   d. when the insurance company does not pay the fee

6. The Truth-in-Lending Act is also known as the:

   a. Consumer Protection Act of 1967

   b. Fair Debt Collection Practice Act

   c. Patient Bankruptcy Protection Act

   d. Accurate Billing and Collection Act

7. The charge slip is also known as the:

   a. ledger

   b. encounter form

   c. day sheet

   d. CMS-1500

8. When a patient files for bankruptcy:

   a. there is little likelihood that the debt can be collected

   b. it is best to close the account and identify the loss

   c. file a proof-of-claim form and provide a copy of the patient's outstanding account to the bankruptcy court

   d. take the account to small claims court

9. In determining how aggressive to be in debt collections, you should consider:

   a. the previous month's billing backlog

   b. production efficiency

   c. the terms of the insured's policy

   d. the value of the dollar owed

LEARNING APPLICATION

Hands-on Activity

Complete the charge slip for Charles Williams' office visit, based on the information below.

Charles Williams, 62 years old, is a new patient of Dr. Winston Lewis at the offices of Drs. Lewis and King. On July 1, 20XX, five days before the patient's birthday, Charles comes to see Dr. Lewis for an appointment with a chief complaint of intermittent, irregular heartbeats or palpitations, dizziness, and chest pain. Dr. Lewis performs a comprehensive physical examination and orders several tests, including an ECG, complete blood count (CBC), and urinalysis with microscopy. The total fee for the office visit and tests is $345—$200 for the physical examination, $75 for the ECG, $25 for the urinalysis, $25 for venipuncture, and $20 for the CBC, which Charles pays for by check at the time of service. Charles is insured by a private carrier, All-American Insurance Company, group #333210, ID number 112-45-9980, which he receives through his employer, High Tech Computer Group. Dr. Lewis asks Ellen Armstrong, CMA (AAMA), to schedule a return appointment in exactly one week to go over the results of Charles's tests. Ellen schedules the appointment and prepares a charge slip for Charles's visit. She refers to his patient information sheet for the correct personal information. Charles Williams lives at 123 Greenside Street, Northborough, OH, 12346.

DATE	PATIENT	SERVICE CODE	FEES CHARGE	PAID CREDITS	ADJ.	BALANCE DUE	PREVIOUS BALANCE	NAME	RECEIPT NO.

THIS IS YOUR RECEIPT _____
AND/OR A STATEMENT OF YOUR ACCOUNT TO DATE _____

PATIENT'S NAME ☒ M ☐ F

ADDRESS

CITY   STATE   ZIP

OFFICE VISITS AND PROCEDURES

99211	EST PT - MINIMAL OV	1		HOSPITAL VISIT	14
99212	EST PT - BRIEF OV	2		EMERGENCY	15
99213	EST PT - INTERMEDIATE OV	3		CONSULTATION	16
99214	EST PT - EXTENDED OV	4	93000	EKG	17
99215	EST PT - COMPREHENSIVE OV	5	93224	ELECTROCARDIOGRAPHIC MONITORING	18
99201	NEW PT - BRIEF OV	6	93307	ECHOCARDIOGRAPHY	19
99202	NEW PT - INTERMEDIATE OV	7	85025	CBC	20
99203	NEW PT - EXTENDED OV	8	81000	URINALYSIS WITH MICROSCOPY	21
99204	NEW PT - COMPLEX OV	9	36415	ROUTINE VENIPUNCTURE	22
99205	NEW PT - COMPREHENSIVE OF	10	71020	RADIOLOGY EXAM-CHEST-2 VIEWS	23
99238	HOSPITAL DISCHARGE	11	30300	REMOVE FOR. BODY-INTRANASAL	24
99025	NEW PT - SURGERY PROC. PRIMARY	12			25
	NURSING HOME VISIT	13			26

RELATIONSHIP   BIRTHDATE

SUBSCRIBER OR POLICY HOLDER

☐ MEDICARE ☐ MEDICAID ☐ BLUE SHIELD ☐ 65-SP.

INSURANCE CARRIER

AGREEMENT #

GROUP #

D - OTHER SERVICES

AUTHORIZATION TO RELEASE INFORMATION: I HEREBY AUTHORIZE THE UNDERSIGNED PHYSICIAN TO RELEASE ANY INFORMATION ACQUIRED IN THE COURSE OF MY EXAMINATION OR TREATMENT.
SIGNED (PATIENT, OR PARENT IF MINOR) _____

DATE _____

NEXT APPOINTMENT _____ AT _____ AM PM

RETURN _____ DAYS _____ WEEKS _____ MONTHS

PLACE OF SERVICE ☒ OFFICE ☐ OTHER _____

DIAGNOSIS OR SYMPTOMS _____

DOCTOR'S SIGNATURE _____

L&K
LEWIS & KING, MD
2501 CENTER STREET
NORTHBOROUGH, OH 12345

03626

Role Play Activity

In groups of three, role play a collection call using the information in Figure 20-6 in your text. One student should role play the medical assistant, one should be the Patient O'Keefe, and the third person should observe and critique. At the conclusion of the role play, the "medical assistant" and "patient" should each discuss how it felt to be the person in that role.

CHAPTER POST-TEST

Perform this test without looking at your book. If an answer is "false," rewrite the sentence to make it true.

1. The Truth-in-Lending Act states:

   a. Providers can charge more than 10% interest on their patient accounts.

   b. Providers can charge interest only if the account is more than four months overdue.

   c. Providers must notify patients in person if interest is to be charged on their accounts.

   d. If the provider and patient agree to an installment plan of more than four payments, the installment charge must be stated in writing.

2. True or False? The best opportunity for collection is within 30 days of the time of service.

   _____

   _____

3. True or False? Large clinics with numerous statements to send out each month will find the cycle billing method to be the most efficient.

   _____

   _____

4. True or False? A collection ratio of 90% is considered a good ratio.

   _____

   _____

SELF-ASSESSMENT

Think about a time or times when you paid a bill late or did not paid it until the following month. Without disclosing too much personal information, answer the following:

1. What was your reason(s)?

   _____

   _____

   _____

   _____

2. Did you receive an overdue notice or a phone call?

   _____

   _____

   _____

   _____

3. Which do you think would be more difficult to receive, the notice or the phone call?

   _____

   _____

   _____

   _____

4. Are you likely to become defensive if the caller or notice has a threatening tone or a more understanding tone? Justify your response.

_____

_____

_____

_____

5. Could the tone of the notice/call leave you feeling good/bad about the event? Explain.

_____

_____

_____

_____

6. Identify ways the situation could have been handled better.

_____

_____

_____

_____

7. Will your experience affect the way you treat people who owe your clinic money?

_____

_____

_____

_____

C H A P T E R **21**

Accounting Practices

CHAPTER PRE-TEST

Perform this test without looking at your book. If an answer is "false," rewrite the sentence to make it true.

1. True or False? Accounts receivable is the amount the provider is owed by patients.

   _____

   _____

2. The purpose of cost analysis is to determine the:

   a. costs of each service

   b. fixed costs

   c. variable costs

   d. total of all of the above

3. True or False? Income statements should show both profits and expenses.

   _____

   _____

4. True or False? The W-4 form shows the employee's withholding allowance.

   _____

   _____

VOCABULARY BUILDER

Misspelled Words

Find the words below that are misspelled; circle them, and correctly spell them in the spaces provided. Then match the vocabulary words to the appropriate definition below.

accounting	cash bases	income statement
accounts payible	check register	libilities
accounts recievable ratio	collection ratio	owner's equity
accrual basis	cost analisys	trial balance
assets	cost ratio	utilazation review
balance sheet	fixed costs	varieble costs

_____
_____
_____

_____   _____
_____

_____   _____
_____

_____   1. Financial statement showing net profit or loss

_____   2. Costs that vary in direct proportion to patient volume

_____   3. Categorizes and records all checks written

_____   4. Formula that measures the speed in which outstanding accounts are paid

_____   5. The purpose of this is to determine the cost of each service

_____   6. An itemized statement of assets, liabilities, financial condition, and owner's equity

_____   7. System of reporting income where income is recognized at the time the money is collected

_____   8. Costs that do not vary in total as the number of patients varies

_____   9. System of monitoring the financial status of a facility and the financial results of its activities, providing information for decision making

_____   10. Debts and other financial obligations for which one is responsible

_____   11. Formula that shows the percentage of outstanding debt collected

_____   12. Properties of value that are owned by a business entity

_____   13. Created by totaling debit balances and credit balances to make sure that total debits equal total credits

_____   14. The amount by which a business's assets exceed the business's liabilities

_____   15. Formula that shows the cost of a procedure or service and helps determine the financial value of maintaining certain services

_____   16. System of reporting income where income is reported at the time charges are generated

_____   17. A review of medical services before they can be performed

LEARNING REVIEW

Short Answer

1. There are a variety of methods used for financial management in the ambulatory care setting. Name three bookkeeping systems that are appropriate for use in a medical office.

_____

_____

2. Medical software packages have the ability to code information obtained in the ambulatory care setting for use in a database. When completing insurance claim forms or generating reports, the software has the capability to include the most common procedural and diagnostic codes. What other kinds of codes can a computerized accounting system generate that will facilitate the billing?

_____

_____

_____

3. The computer can also be used in the preparation of financial documents. Name four financial documents.

_____

_____

4. Name three ways computer service bureaus handle accounts from medical facilities.

_____

_____

_____

_____

_____

5. Identify at least four steps to take to reduce the chance of embezzlement.

_____

_____

_____

_____

_____

6. To protect the practice from financial loss, providers can purchase fidelity bonds. Name and describe the three kinds of bonds. Place an X in front of the one that offers the most assurance.

   1. _____   _____

   2. _____   _____

   3. _____   _____

7. How might the office manager use data from the budget sheet?

_____

_____

_____

8. Why is it important to implement and track budgets for specific categories of income and expense in the ambulatory care setting?

_____

_____

_____

Matching I

Match the appropriate noncomputerized bookkeeping system to the following duties performed by the medical assistant.

A. Single-entry

B. Pegboard

C. Double-entry

_____ 1. Office manager Walter Seals was responsible for implementing a computer system at Inner City Health Care. Before the computerized accounting program was put into effect, the urgent care center relied on a manual system of checks and balances that allowed the provider-employers to keep a firm hold on the relation between the facility's assets and the sum of liabilities and net worth.

_____ 2. During a temporary one-week down period in the computer system at the offices of Drs. Lewis and King while a system upgrade is installed, administrative medical assistant Ellen Armstrong completes each day's financial transactions in a daily journal, then transfers this information to the ledger through the posting process. The information will be entered into the computer once the system is up and running again.

_____ 3. When the patient returns the charge slip to the reception desk after an examination, medical assistant Karen Ritter carefully replaces and lines up the charge slip with the patient's name on the day sheet, then correctly inserts the ledger card under the last page of the charge slip. She proceeds to enter the total charges due and any patient payments.

Fixed and Variable Costs Exercise

Fixed costs are expenses that do not vary in total as the number of patients seen by the medical practice grows or shrinks. Variable costs are expenses that are directly affected by patient volume. From the list below, identify expenses that qualify as fixed costs (FC) and those that are variable costs (VC).

_____ 1. Interpreting laboratory test results

_____ 2. Annual depreciation of the cost of an automatic electrocardiograph (ECG) machine

_____ 3. Medical benefits for the office staff

_____ 4. Purchase of reagent test strips for urinalysis

_____ 5. Magazine subscriptions for the facility reception area

_____ 6. Monthly telephone expenses

_____ 7. Medical journal subscriptions for the providers

_____ 8. Purchase of a HemoCue blood glucose system

_____ 9. Printing cost of a patient education brochure

_____ 10. Purchase of open-shelf lateral files

_____ 11. Adding a new position, such as a clinical medical assistant, to the office staff

_____ 12. Property taxes on the medical facility building and grounds

_____ 13. The monthly cost of janitorial services

_____ 14. Purchase of disposable needle-syringe units

_____ 15. Disposable paper gowns for patient examinations

CERTIFICATION REVIEW

These questions are designed to mimic the certification examination. Select the best response.

1. The system that is based on the accounting principle that assets equal liabilities plus owner's equity is the:

   a. single-entry system

   b. double-entry system

   c. standard of billing services bureaus

   d. accounts receivable accounting principles

2. Of the following statements, which is false?

   a. Double-entry bookkeeping is expensive.

   b. Double-entry bookkeeping is accurate.

   c. Double-entry bookkeeping is more time consuming.

   d. Double-entry bookkeeping has checks and balances in place.

3. Owner's equity is *not* the same as:

   a. net worth

   b. proprietorship

   c. capital

   d. accounts payable

4. Bonds may be purchased to protect the practice from:

   a. embezzlement

   b. financial loss

   c. malpractice suits

   d. a. and b.

   e. all of the above

5. A total practice management system has the ability to:

   a. process insurance claims electronically

   b. manage payroll and purchases

   c. generate financial records

   d. All of the above

6. Computerization of medical facilities has increased because of:

   a. emphasis being placed on the accurate documentation of medical records

   b. patient load

   c. increase in managed care plans

   d. a. and c.

7. The trial balance is created by:

    a. collecting data from the current year and previous year and converting them into a ratio

    b. totaling debit balances and credit balances to confirm that total debits equal total credits

    c. reporting outside revenue sources and overhead expenses

    d. recording two sets of entries, such as increase in assets and increase in liabilities

8. Providers should purchase fidelity bonds because they:

    a. are worth the price

    b. provide a sense of security

    c. lessen the chances of embezzlement

    d. will reimburse the practice for any monetary loss caused by the practice's employees

9. A proper contract should be negotiated and signed with any computer and billing service bureau because it:

    a. is considered a legal document

    b. ensures confidentiality and strict privacy of patient information

    c. is in compliance with HIPAA

    d. b. and c.

10. Financial records should provide the following at all times:

    a. salaries earned by providers and staff

    b. amount earned, owed, and collected within a given period

    c. where expenses were incurred in a given period

    d. b. and c.

11. A hospital cost report for Medicare is a part of:

    a. financial accounting

    b. managerial accounting

    c. cost accounting

    d. cost analysis

12. Examples of variable costs include all of the following *except:*

    a. clinical supplies

    b. equipment costs

    c. depreciation

    d. laboratory procedures

13. The accounts receivable trial balance:

    a. tells you how much the practice owes to creditors

    b. shows any problems between the daily journal and the ledger

    c. tracks all disbursements and compares the total with the purchases

    d. uses an NCR transfer strip to copy pertinent information

14. Calculating and reviewing costs provide ambulatory care settings with:

    a. data to set fees

    b. monitoring of the practice's performance

    c. offline batch processing

    d. a. and b.

LEARNING APPLICATION

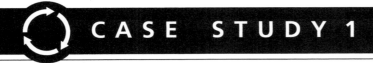
CASE STUDY 1

When the offices of Drs. Lewis and King agreed to accept individuals covered by a large managed care organization, the decision of the provider-owners was based on a complete financial analysis and projection of the expected effects the new patient load would have on the medical practice. As a result, the group practice added a second office manager and a new clinical medical assistant to the existing staff.

CASE STUDY REVIEW QUESTIONS

1. As Drs. Lewis and King absorb the new managed care patients into the practice, what can the provider-owners do to determine whether their financial analysis and projection were accurate?

    _____

    _____

    _____

2. Once the practice has assembled financial data on the effects of the new patient load, how will these data be used?

    _____

    _____

    _____

    _____

    _____

3. What beneficial effects might the addition of a clinical medical assistant have on the medical practice?

    _____

    _____

    _____

    _____

    _____

CASE STUDY 2

A group practice of radiologists charges $225 for a routine mammogram. Total expenses related to the mammogram procedure equal $30,000 per month, and the practice performs a monthly average of 200 mammograms.

CASE STUDY REVIEW QUESTIONS

1. What is the average cost ratio for the mammogram procedure? Show your calculations in the space provided.

_____

_____

2. Given the cost to patients for the mammogram procedure, is the group practice making a profit or loss on performing mammograms? What amount is the profit or loss per procedure? What amount is the profit or loss for the entire month?

_____

_____

_____

Hands-on Activities

1. At the offices of Drs. Lewis and King, the total accounts receivable at the end of May is $100,000 and the monthly receipts total is $75,000; the total accounts receivable at the end of June is $82,000 and the monthly receipts total is $31,000; the total accounts receivable at the end of July is $86,000 and the monthly receipts total is $20,000; the total accounts receivable at the end of August is $93,000 and the monthly receipts total is $45,000. What is the accounts receivable ratio for each month? Show your calculations in the space provided. Which month has the healthiest accounts receivable ratio? Why?

   May: _____   July: _____

   June: _____   August: _____

_____

_____

_____

2. For the month of September, receipts at the offices of Drs. Lewis and King totaled $35,000. The Medicare/Medicaid adjustment for the month was $1,750, and the managed care adjustment was $4,500. Total charges for the month of September equaled $53,000. What is the collection ratio for the month of September? Show your calculation in the space provided.

_____

_____

3. For the month of October, receipts at the offices of Drs. Lewis and King totaled $41,000. The Medicare/Medicaid adjustment for the month was $2,000, the Worker's Compensation adjustment was $750, and the managed care adjustment was $4,700. Total charges for October equaled $55,000. What is the collection ratio for the month of October? Show your calculation in the space provided.

_____

_____

4. Income statements reveal the cumulative profit and total expenses for each month.Monthly income and expenses are then added to arrive at year-to-date totals, which are compared with the annual budget for particular income and expense categories. Use the following information to complete the expense analysis table for the first quarter office expense costs of the offices of Drs. Lewis and King. The total office expense budget for the year is $20,000 divided evenly per quarter.

Telephone expenses
January $323.46
February $425.93
March $393.87

Postage and mail expenses
January $725.45
February $550.90
March $601.33

Office supply expenses
January $1,200.62
February $325.45
March $446.26

Yearly budget
Telephone expenses $4,000
Postage and mail expenses $8,000
Office supply expenses $8,000

Office Expenses	January	February	March	Year to Date	Budget for Year
Telephone	_____	_____	_____	_____	_____
Postage	_____	_____	_____	_____	_____
Office supplies	_____	_____	_____	_____	_____
TOTALS	_____	_____	_____	_____	_____

CHAPTER POST-TEST

Perform this test without looking at your book. If an answer is "false," rewrite the sentence to make it true.

1. True or False? Accounts payable is the amount the provider is owed by patients.

_____

_____

2. The purpose of cost analysis is to:

a. determine the costs of each service

b. determine the fixed costs

c. determine the variable costs

d. determine the total of all of the above

3. True or False? Both profits and expenses should be shown on income statements.

_____

_____

4. True or False? Employees' withholding allowance is recorded on the W-4 form.

_____

_____

SELF-ASSESSMENT

Personal finances, as well as the finances of businesses such as ambulatory care settings, require careful planning, management, and budgeting. You can use the systems of business financial management to gain insights into your personal spending patterns and to help develop and fine-tune smart financial habits and attitudes. For each statement, circle the response that best describes you.

1. I think saving money is:

   a. important; I make every effort to put away a sum of money as savings on a regular basis.

   b. great if you can find a way; I would like to save, but I have trouble finding ways to do it.

   c. not important right now; I have too many expenses—what I really need is a loan!

2. When planning a large purchase, such as a computer or a car, I:

   a. set a limit for spending and affordable installment payments and stick to it.

   b. have a rough idea of what I can afford, but do not do any advance planning.

   c. try to buy what I want and think about paying for it later.

3. When considering monthly personal income and expenses, I:

   a. know exactly how much money is coming in and how much is going out to pay bills.

   b. know I can cover my bills but do not keep track of exactly how much I make or spend.

   c. hope for the best, and if I fall short—charge it!

4. When I have extra money, I:

   a. save one-third, use one-third to pay off debts, and use the last third on a special purchase.

   b. save half or use it to pay off debts and spend the other half on a special purchase.

   c. spend it all on a special purchase.

5. My checkbook is:

   a. always balanced.

   b. sometimes balanced.

   c. rarely balanced.

6. When choosing a bank for my savings or checking, I:

   a. research interest rates, features, funds, and services carefully to find the best deal.

   b. choose the bank that pays the highest interest rate.

   c. just pick whatever is most convenient; banks are all the same.

7. I think planning for retirement is:

    a. a priority now; the sooner you start saving, the more your money grows!

    b. important but not the most essential financial responsibility I have right now.

    c. not something I think about now—that is too far away; who can predict the future?

8. People think of me as someone who:

    a. pays attention to detail and is neat and organized.

    b. always manages to get the job done at the last minute.

    c. struggles to keep up with routine or repetitive tasks.

9. I think analyzing financial data is:

    a. a smart way to assess current spending patterns and guide future spending.

    b. a great thing to do if you have enough time and willpower.

    c. a waste of time; besides, I just do not want to know.

10. I am the kind of person who:

    a. sets short- and long-term financial goals for income and spending and works toward implementing them in a responsible way.

    b. has short- and long-term financial goals but cannot get around to planning for them.

    c. makes financial decisions on a day-to-day basis; it is enough to deal with one day at a time.

Scoring: If your answers were mostly A responses, congratulations! You have developed a financially responsible outlook and good record-keeping habits. If your responses were mostly Bs, you are thinking about financial realities and recognize the importance of a strong financial awareness. Focus on specifics where you can improve your financial skills. If your responses were mostly Cs, you need to work on achieving good personal financial habits. Start working on your record-keeping skills by taking the plunge and keeping a weekly journal of expenses to see where your money goes!

C H A P T E R **2 2**

The Medical Assistant as Office Manager

CHAPTER PRE-TEST

Perform this test without looking at your book. If an answer is "false," rewrite the sentence to make it true.

1. True or False? Teamwork results in getting more accomplished with the resources available.

_____

_____

2. True or False? Office managers do not need effective communication skills.

_____

_____

3. True or False? It is not necessary to update the office procedures manual.

_____

_____

4. True or False? Minutes should be sent only to the team members who attended the meeting.

_____

_____

5. True or False? When working with an externing student, each step should be explained together with the rationale.

_____

_____

6. True or False? Office managers need to be able to accept and offer criticism constructively.

_____

_____

7. True or False? The office manager will always serve as the human resources director.

_____

_____

VOCABULARY BUILDER

Misspelled Words

Find the words listed below that are misspelled; circle them, and correctly spell them in the spaces provided. Then insert the correct vocabulary terms beside the sentences that follow.

agenda	"going bare"	practicum
ancilliary services	itinerary	procedures manual
benchmarking	liability	professional liability insurance
benefits	marketing	risk management
bond	minutes	teamwork
embezzel	negligance	work statement
externs		

_____   _____   _____

_____

_____

_____

_____

_____

_____

_____

_____

_____

_____

_____

_____

1. Professional occupational companies hired to complete a specific job such as janitorial services, laundry, or disposal of hazardous materials

2. The situation of a provider who does not carry insurance to protect the provider's assets in the event of a liability claim

3. Making a comparison between different organizations relative to how they accomplish tasks, remunerate employees, and so on

4. Designed to protect assets in the event a liability claim is filed and awarded

5. A written record of topics discussed and actions taken during meeting sessions

6. This provides a concise description of the work you plan to accomplish

7. A binding agreement with an employee ensuring recovery of financial loss should funds be stolen or embezzled

8. A printed list of topics to be discussed during a meeting

9. The process by which the provider of services makes the consumer aware of the scope and quality of those services. Examples might include public relations, brochures, patient education seminars, and newsletters.

10. Involves persons synergistically working together

11. A transitional stage providing an opportunity to apply theory learned in the classroom to a health care setting through practical, hands-on experience

12. Remuneration that is in addition to a salary

13. To appropriate fraudulently for one's own use

14. Involves the identification, analysis, and treatment of risks within the medical office or facility

_____   15. Performing an act that a reasonable and prudent provider would not perform.

_____   16. Provides detailed information relative to the performance of tasks within the facility in which one is employed

_____   17. A detailed plan for a proposed trip

LEARNING REVIEW

Short Answer

1. The office manager of a medical office or ambulatory care facility can have many varied responsibilities based on individual facility needs. What are five duties that are the responsibility of the office manager in a health care setting?

_____

_____

_____

_____

_____

_____

_____

_____

_____

2. What are five attributes needed to perform as a quality manager in any office setting?

_____

_____

_____

3. What is the difference between authoritarian and participatory management styles?

_____

_____

_____

_____

_____

4. What does "management by walking around" mean, and why would it be useful in a medical office setting?

_____

_____

_____

5. The table below discusses some of the common risks for medical offices, as well as risk control measures for each one. Fill in any missing information.

Risk	Risk Control Measures
_____	Train various employees to assume other duties and perform them when an employee is ill, on vacation, etc.
Failure of a supplier or contractor	_____ _____ _____ _____ _____
_____	Have protocols in place for handling this situation and make patients aware of the protocols; notify patients immediately if confidential information is disclosed and work with them toward resolution.
Computer failure	_____ _____ _____ _____ _____
_____	Continually review safety procedures; conduct safety surveys; always carry liability insurance; complete an Incident Report to signal risk manager to implement existing protocols to minimize risk

6. Define harassment in the workplace.

_____

_____

_____

_____

7. List the steps that a manager should take if he or she is made aware of harassment in the medical office.

_____

_____

_____

_____

_____

8. Why do some employers put new employees on probation? What is the usual length of an employee's probationary period?

_____

_____

_____

_____

Ordering Activity

All administrative and clinical supplies and equipment in the facility must be inventoried. The following tasks are performed when new supplies and/or equipment are received. Put the tasks steps in the correct order, from 1 to 5.

_____ A. Unpack each item, checking against the packing slip.

_____ B. Write the date the shipment was received and who verified it.

_____ C. Stock each item appropriately.

_____ D. Verify that no items have been substituted or backordered.

_____ E. Find the packing slip listing the items ordered.

Matching

Most marketing tools used in a medical environment provide educational and office services information to patients, potential patients, and the local community. Match the following marketing tools with their potential use in the ambulatory care facility setting.

A. Seminars
B. Brochures
C. Newsletters
D. Press releases
E. Special events

_____ 1. These are used for announcing new equipment, new staff, expanded or remodeled office space, and so on.

_____ 2. These typically come in two types—patient education and office services—and present a professional image of the ambulatory care setting.

_____ 3. These provide an effective way to join with other community organizations to promote wellness.

_____ 4. These can educate patients and provide goodwill in the community. All facility staff can work as a team to organize these.

_____ 5. These can include a wide range of information from health-related topics to staff introductions to insurance updates. They may form the nucleus of a marketing program.

CERTIFICATION REVIEW

These questions are designed to mimic the certification examination. Select the best response.

1. There is a direct correlation between a person's management style and his or her:

   a. technical expertise

   b. educational level

   c. personality

   d. salary

2. Most conflicts occur between employees and supervisors or providers because of:

   a. attitude

   b. poor communication

   c. a misunderstanding

   d. b. and c.

3. The person who applies the team-oriented management style is often comfortable with:

   a. teaching and coaching

   b. building, constructing, and modeling

   c. ideas, information, and data

   d. all of the above

4. A comprehensive safety program is essential to:

   a. marketing functions

   b. team building

   c. risk management

   d. equipment and supply maintenance

5. Leadership for the twenty-first century includes components of flexibility, mentoring, and:

   a. networking

   b. domination

   c. hierarchy

   d. rigidity

6. A rule that defines almost all of the ethical qualities of a manager is:

   a. Murphy's law

   b. the Rule of Nines

   c. the Golden Rule

   d. none of the above

7. The _____ management style is based on the premise that the worker is capable and wants to do a good job.

   a. walking around

   b. participatory

   c. risk

   d. authoritarian

8. The most significant task(s) of the team leader or office manager is (are):

   a. getting the team members to understand and support the specifics of the problem they are asked to solve

   b. enabling the team to develop their own work statement where they will assume ownership of the goals and objectives

   c. establishing a timetable for achieving results and identifying the standards that must be maintained

   d. all of the above

9. The documentation of policies and procedures that make up the office HIPAA manual should be:

   a. filed in a locked cabinet

   b. kept for six years, even though wording has been changed or has been eliminated

   c. made available for all employees

   d. b. and c.

10. If malpractice litigation should occur, the best protocol to follow is to:

    a. be honest with the patients and insurance carriers

    b. let the HR person handle the situation

    c. notify the provider

    d. not get involved

LEARNING APPLICATION

Time Management Activity

To practice your time management skills, make a to-do list for tomorrow or the upcoming weekend. Prioritize the list by importance.

CASE STUDY

Office manager Shirley Brooks is responsible for the preparation and distribution of payroll checks at the offices of Drs. Lewis and King. Because the group practice is in the process of upgrading the computer system to accommodate a recent influx of new patients, Shirley is temporarily preparing the payroll using the manual write-it-once bookkeeping system. She is careful to consult payroll records for each employee, which include the employee's name, address, telephone number, and Social Security number; number of exemptions claimed on the W-4 form; gross salary; deductions withheld for all taxes, including Social Security, federal, state, local unemployment and disability; and date of employment.

CASE STUDY REVIEW QUESTIONS

1. As Shirley writes out the payroll check for Audrey Jones, CMA (AAMA), what information should be included on the paycheck stub?

   _____

   _____

   _____

   _____

   _____

   _____

2. What must the provider's office have to process payroll?

   _____

   _____

   _____

3. What responsibility does the office manager have with regard to the confidentiality of payroll records? How might employees' rights to privacy be maintained?

   _____

   _____

   _____

   _____

   _____

   _____

CHAPTER POST-TEST

Perform this test without looking at your book. If an answer is "false," rewrite the sentence to make it true.

1. True or False? Teamwork results in getting less accomplished with the resources available.

   _____

   _____

2. True or False? Office managers need effective communication skills.

   _____

   _____

3. True or False? It is necessary to update the office procedures manual.

   _____

   _____

4. True or False? Minutes should be sent to all team members, not just those who attended the meeting.

   _____

   _____

5. True or False? When working with externing students, each step does not need to be explained together with the rationale, because they already have training.

   _____

   _____

6. True or False? Office managers need to be able to offer criticism constructively, but they should not have to accept criticism.

   _____

   _____

7. True or False? The person who is the office manager is never the human resources director.

   _____

   _____

SELF-ASSESSMENT

Put yourself in the place of the office manager.

1. What type of management style do you think you are the most comfortable with?

   _____

   _____

   _____

   _____

2. Carefully read about each type of style and explain why you think you are that type.

_____

_____

_____

_____

3. What skills will come naturally to you?

_____

_____

_____

_____

4. What skills will you have to work on the most?

_____

_____

_____

_____

C H A P T E R **23**

The Medical Assistant as Human Resources Manager

CHAPTER PRE-TEST

Perform this test without looking at your book. If an answer is "false," rewrite the sentence to make it true.

1. Which of the following is *not* a function of the human resources (HR) manager?

   a. Creating and updating a policy manual

   b. Recruiting and hiring office personnel

   c. Orienting new personnel

   d. Training new personnel

2. True or False? Wage and salary policies should be in writing.

   _____

   _____

3. True or False? A policy manual should contain daily step-by-step instructions.

   _____

   _____

4. True or False? Job descriptions are not always useful because they change so often.

   _____

   _____

5. True or False? All job applicants should be interviewed.

   _____

   _____

6. True or False? It is acceptable to ask job applicants about the last place they worked and a conflict they had there.

   _____

   _____

7. True or False? References are usually checked after the first interview.

_____

_____

8. True or False? The HR manager is responsible for dismissing employees.

_____

_____

9. True or False? Employees have a right to review their personnel files at any time.

_____

_____

10. True or False? Employers have the right to refuse to allow full-time employees to go on jury duty.

_____

_____

VOCABULARY BUILDER

Misspelled Words

Find the words listed below that are misspelled; circle them, and correctly spell them in the spaces provided. Then, insert the correct vocabulary terms into the following sentences.

exit interveiw	letter of referance	overtime
involuntary dismisal	letter of resignation	probation
job desciption	menter	résumés

_____   _____   _____

_____   _____

1. Because of an unexpected staffing shortfall, Audrey Jones, CMA (AAMA), has volunteered to work _____ this week. She will receive 1½ times the regular rate of pay for hours above her regular 40-hour week.

2. An _____ has been scheduled for administrative/clinical medical assistant Liz Corbin before she leaves the clinic to continue her education. This session will give Liz an opportunity to provide her positive and negative opinions of the position and the facility.

3. Office manager Marilyn Johnson has received a _____ from the former instructor of a current job applicant describing the applicant's performance, attitude, and qualifications.

4. The violation of office policies at Inner City Health Care led to the _____ of one of the part-time employees.

5. Liz Corbin, CMA (AAMA), submitted a _____ to her current employer when she decided to leave her present position to return to school to pursue an advanced degree.

6. Office manager Marilyn Johnson will inform all of the job applicants that they will be on _____ for their first three months on the job. During this period, the employee and supervisory personnel can determine if the environment and the position are satisfactory for the employee.

7. Office manager Jane O'Hara, updating the employee manual, includes a _____ for every position in the office, which details tasks, duties, and responsibilities.

8. Administrative medical assistant Ellen Armstrong looks upon office manager Marilyn Johnson as her _____, since Marilyn has been instrumental in Ellen's training, coaching, and guidance in her newly acquired position.

LEARNING REVIEW

Short Answer

1. The manual that identifies clear guidelines and directions required of all employees is known as the policy manual. What are four topics that would be included in a policy manual regardless of the size of the practice identified in this chapter?

   _____

   _____

   _____

2. Office manager Marilyn Johnson has the responsibility of dismissing an employee for a serious violation of office policies. From the list below, select key points to keep in mind when dismissal is necessary by circling the letters of the statements that apply.

   a. Have employee pack his or her belongings from desk.

   b. The dismissal should be made in private.

   c. Take no longer than 20 minutes for the dismissal.

   d. Be direct, firm, and to the point in identifying reasons.

   e. Explain terms of dismissal (keys, clearing out area, final paperwork).

   f. Do not listen to the employee's opinion and emotions.

   g. If he or she insists, allow the employee to finish the work of the day.

   h. Do not engage in an in-depth discussion of performance.

3. Compare and contrast voluntary and involuntary separation.

   _____

   _____

   _____

   _____

   _____

   _____

4. The job description must have enough information to provide both the supervisor and the employee with a clear outline of what the job entails. Name four items that must be included in a job description.

   _____

   _____

   _____

5. The interview worksheet is an excellent tool to make certain that the interviews with each candidate are fair and equitable. Provide six items that should be included on any interview worksheet.

   _____

   _____

   _____

   _____

   _____

CERTIFICATION REVIEW

These questions are designed to mimic the certification examination. Select the best response.

1. A salary review is:

   a. usually conducted at the beginning of the new year

   b. virtually the same as the performance review

   c. conducted on the anniversary date of hire

   d. normally done every three years

2. Questions regarding drug use, arrest records, and medical history during an interview are:

   a. appropriate

   b. inappropriate

   c. illegal

   d. none of the above

3. Title VII of the Civil Rights Act addresses:

   a. overtime pay

   b. discrimination based on race, age, and sex

   c. hiring and firing practices

   d. sexual harassment

4. When a candidate accepts a position, the HR manager should write a letter outlining the specifics of the job. This letter is called a:

   a. confirmation letter

   b. congratulatory letter

   c. recommendation letter

   d. reference letter

5. A person with AIDS who satisfies the necessary skills for a job and has the experience and education required will be protected from discrimination by:

   a. OSHA

   b. CLIA

   c. AAMA

   d. ADA

6. A job description should be reviewed and updated:

   a. every 2 years

   b. every 90 days

   c. every year

   d. every 5 years

7. Voluntary separation usually occurs when:

    a. advancing to another position

    b. there is a violation of office policies

    c. the employee is relocating

    d. a. and c.

8. Verifying that all employees are authorized to work is done by

    a. asking for verbal clarification

    b. having the candidate complete an I-9 form

    c. having the candidate provide a notarized statement

    d. having the candidate fill out an attestation form

9. What documents should be included in the personnel file? *(circle all that apply)*

    a. Application

    b. Formal review

    c. Awards

    d. Employee handbook

10. What act was established to prevent injuries and illnesses resulting from unsafe and unhealthy working conditions?

    a. Americans with Disabilities Act

    b. Civil Rights Act

    c. OSHA

    d. Equal Pay Act

LEARNING APPLICATION

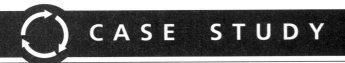

CASE STUDY

Since the offices of Drs. Lewis and King have expanded to cover a rapidly growing patient load, including the hiring of a co–office manager and a new clinical medical assistant, the work pace has been hectic, but challenging. At the suggestion of Dr. Lewis, the office managers decide to hold a staff meeting to talk about ways to keep the lines of communication open and to process the many changes occurring at the growing medical practice. Marilyn Johnson and Shirley Brooks encourage staff to be vocal with their feedback, suggestions, and concerns.

CASE STUDY REVIEW QUESTIONS

1. What other techniques can the office managers use to prevent or solve conflicts in the workplace during the period of growth and transition?

   _____

   _____

   _____

   _____

   _____

   _____

   _____

   _____

2. Why is effective communication one of the most important goals of the HR manager?

   _____

   _____

   _____

CHAPTER POST-TEST

Perform this test without looking at your book. If an answer is "false," rewrite the sentence to make it true.

1. Which of the following are functions of the HR manager? *(Circle all that apply)*

   a. Creating and updating a policy manual

   b. Training new personnel

   c. Recruiting and hiring office personnel

   d. Orienting new personnel

2. True or False? Wage and salary policies need not be in writing as long as both parties agree.

   _____

   _____

3. True or False? A policy manual should contain general policies and practices of the office.

   _____

   _____

4. True or False? Job descriptions are always useful and should be clearly written.

   _____

   _____

5. True or False? Only qualified job applicants should be interviewed.

   _____

   _____

6. True or False? It is good to ask job applicants about conflicts they have had and how they solved them.

   _____

   _____

7. True or False? References are usually checked before the first interview.

   _____

   _____

8. True or False? The HR manager is responsible for the exit interview, but usually not for dismissing employees.

   _____

   _____

9. True or False? Employees do not have the right to review their personnel files unless requested by an attorney.

   _____

   _____

10. True or False? Employers cannot condemn or discriminate against a full-time employee who is on jury duty.

    _____

    _____

SELF-ASSESSMENT

1. If you were put into the position of hiring a new employee, what attributes would you be looking for?

   a. Make a list of the technical skills your new employee would need.

   _____

   _____

   b. Make a list of the affective (behavior) skills your new employee would need, including a positive attitude, a good work ethic, and so forth.

   _____

   _____

   _____

   _____

   c. Determine how you could measure the technical skills you listed.

   _____

   _____

   _____

   d. Determine how you could quantify the affective (behavior) skills you listed in item b. above. How could you determine those qualities?

   _____

   _____

   _____

   e. Which is more difficult to measure: technical or behavioral qualities? Which is more difficult to train?

   _____

   _____

2. When you interview for a job, what technical and behavioral skills on your lists will you need to improve on?

   _____

   _____

C H A P T E R **2 4**

Preparing for Medical Assisting Credentials

CHAPTER PRE-TEST

Perform this test without looking at your book. If an answer is "false," rewrite the sentence to make it true.

1. True or False? A registered medical assistant (RMA) and a certified medical assistant (CMA [AAMA]) have the same bylaws and creed.

   _____

   _____

2. True or False? A CMA (AAMA) may work only in the state in which the credentials were received.

   _____

   _____

3. True or False? Three major areas included in the RMA examination are clinical, administrative, and general medical knowledge.

   _____

   _____

4. True or False? Medical assistants may be trained on the job; however, providers recognize that their offices operate much more efficiently and effectively with professionally trained and formally educated personnel.

   _____

   _____

5. True or False? On meeting CMA recertification requirements, the applicant will receive a new certificate.

   _____

   _____

6. True or False? Once a student has become a member of AAMA, he or she may stay at the student rate for one year after graduation.

   _____

   _____

7. True or False? The National Healthcare Association (NHA) does not offer continuing education programs and does not encourage recertification.

_____

_____

8. True or False? Retaking the RMA examination is not an option for reinstatement or recertification.

_____

_____

VOCABULARY BUILDER

Matching

Match each correct vocabulary term to the aspect of the certification process that best describes it.

_____ 1. Certification examination

_____ 2. Certified medical assistant (CMA [AAMA])

_____ 3. Continuing education units (CEUs)

_____ 4. Certified clinical medical assistant (CCMA)

_____ 5. Recertification

_____ 6. Registered medical assistant (RMA)

_____ 7. Task Force for Test Construction

A. Method for earning points toward recertification

B. A standardized means of evaluating medical assistant competency

C. Maintaining current CMA (AAMA) status

D. Credential awarded for successfully passing the AAMA certification examination

E. Committee of professionals whose responsibility is to update the CMA (AAMA) examination annually to reflect changes in medical assistants' responsibilities and to include new developments in medical knowledge and technology

F. Credential awarded for successfully passing the AMT examination

G. One of the credentials awarded for passing the National Healthcare Association exam

LEARNING REVIEW

Short Answer

1. The AAMA certification examination is a comprehensive test of the knowledge based on tasks performed in today's medical office. The test is updated annually to include the latest changes in medical assistants' daily responsibilities. In addition, the updates include the latest developments in medical knowledge and technology. Name the three major areas tested in the AAMA certification examination and describe what each includes.

_____

_____

_____

_____

_____

_____

_____

2. What are the addresses, telephone numbers, and Web sites for obtaining applications for the certification examinations of the AAMA, AMT, and NHA?

AAMA   _____

   _____

   _____

AMT   _____

   _____

   _____

NHA   _____

   _____

   _____

3. To keep their CMA (AAMA) credentials current, how often are individuals required to recertify? How many continuing education units (CEUs) are necessary to recertify?

_____

_____

_____

4. In addition to the RMA credential, what is the credential that the AMT offers for those who primarily want to be employed in the front office of provider offices, clinics, or hospitals?

_____

_____

5. List the criteria an applicant must possess for taking the NHA certification exam.

_____

_____

_____

_____

_____

CERTIFICATION REVIEW

These questions are designed to mimic the certification examination. Select the best response.

1. General medical assisting knowledge on the AMT certification examination includes anatomy and physiology, medical terminology, and:

   a. insurance and billing

   b. medical ethics

   c. bookkeeping and filing

   d. first aid

2. The AMT registration exam consists of:

   a. 300 multiple choice questions

   b. 250 multiple choice questions

   c. 200–210 four-option multiple choice questions

   d. 500 multiple choice questions

3. A total of how many questions are on the CMA (AAMA) certification examination?

   a. 100

   b. 200

   c. 1,000

   d. It varies year to year.

4. How often does an RMA need to recertify?

   a. Every year

   b. Every 6 years

   c. Every 5 years

   d. Every 3 years

5. A total of how many CEUs are required to recertify the CMA (AAMA) credential?

   a. 45

   b. 60

   c. 100

   d. 120

6. When recertifying through the AAMA, a minimum of _____ points is required in each of the three categories. The remaining _____ points may be accumulated in any of the three content areas or from any combination of the three categories.

   a. 15, 60

   b. 20, 40

   c. 10, 30

   d. 30, 60

7. The purpose of certification is that it:

   a. acknowledges that you are a professional with standard entry-level knowledge and skills

   b. builds your personal self-esteem and confidence in knowing that you can do the job asked of you

   c. helps in your career advancement and compensation

   d. All of the above

LEARNING APPLICATION

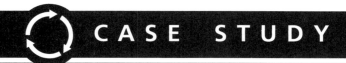

CASE STUDY

Michele Lucas is performing her practicum at Inner City Health Care under the direction of office manager Jane O'Hara. Michele has purchased a certification review study guide and has taken the sample 120-question certification examination available from the AAMA. From her studies, she has determined that she needs more work in the area of collections and insurance processing. Part-time administrative medical assistant Karen Ritter is responsible for these duties at Inner City Health Care, under Jane's supervision.

CASE STUDY REVIEW QUESTIONS

1. How can Michele use her practicum experience to help her concentrate on improving her skills in the area of collections and insurance processing?

   _____

   _____

   _____

   _____

   _____

   _____

2. What are your own personal strengths and weaknesses in preparing for a certification examination through AAMA, AMT, or NHA? What can you do to improve your areas of weakness?

   _____

   _____

   _____

CHAPTER POST-TEST

Perform this test without looking at your book. If an answer is "false," rewrite the sentence to make it true.

1. True or False? An RMA and a CMA (AAMA) have different bylaws and creeds.

   _____

   _____

2. True or False? A CMA (AAMA) has a national credential, so he or she may work in any state.

   _____

   _____

3. True or False? Three major areas included in the AMT's RMA examination are clinical, administrative, and general.

   _____

   _____

4. True or False? Providers recognize that their offices operate much more efficiently and effectively with professionally trained and formally educated personnel such as medical assistants.

_____

_____

5. True or False? Upon meeting recertification requirements, applicants receive an identification card which will indicate the year of recertification and the expiration date.

_____

_____

6. True or False? Once students have become members of AAMA, they may stay at the student rate for two years after graduation.

_____

_____

7. True or False? The NHA encourages recertification and offers CE programs.

_____

_____

8. True or False? Retaking the RMA examination is an option for reinstatement or recertification.

_____

_____

SELF-ASSESSMENT

1. Think of two different places where you could get continuing education credits.

   a. Investigate each one.

   b. Write a paragraph on the benefits and disadvantages of each method for you in your lifestyle.

2. Find out when and where your local chapter meetings are held.

   a. Attend a meeting with a classmate.

   b. Discuss what you learned from the meeting.

3. What can you do to prepare for the national certification examination?

   a. Write a plan in which you determine how much time you have to prepare and what you will accomplish each week/month in preparation.

   b. Make a calendar showing the steps toward your examination date.

   c. Try to stick with the plan as you progress closer to the examination date.

C H A P T E R **2 5**

Employment Strategies

CHAPTER PRE-TEST

Perform this test without looking at your book. If an answer is "false," rewrite the sentence to make it true.

1. True or False? Positive thinking is one of the primary keys to success in planning your career and doing your job search.

   _____

   _____

2. True or False? It would be beneficial to begin your job search by networking with students who have graduated before you and are now successfully employed.

   _____

   _____

3. True or False? Poor appearance is a reason for employers not to hire a job seeker.

   _____

   _____

4. True or False? Employers like it when you know it all. They appreciate it when you do not ask questions.

   _____

   _____

5. True or False? You should never expect to receive a job from an office where you are an extern.

   _____

   _____

6. True or False? When filling out an application, it is acceptable to leave answers blank or write "see résumé."

   _____

   _____

7. True or False? You should always plan ahead and have all your information with you when picking up an application, just in case you are asked to fill it out right there.

   _____

   _____

VOCABULARY BUILDER

Misspelled Words

Find the words listed below that are misspelled; circle them, and correctly spell them in the spaces provided. Then match each correct vocabulary term to the aspect of the job-seeking process that best describes it.

accomplishment statement

application form

bullat point

carreer objective

contact tracker

cover letter

cronological résumé

functional résumé

interview

power verbs

refrences

résumé

targeted résumé

_____

_____

_____

_____

_____

_____

1. Expresses your career goal and the position for which you are applying

2. Résumé format used to highlight specialty areas of accomplishments and strengths

3. A form devised by a prospective employer to collect information relative to qualifications, education, and experience in employment

4. Individuals who have known or worked with you long enough to make an honest assessment and recommendation regarding your background history

5. Résumé format used when focusing on a clear, specific job

6. A statement that begins with a power verb and gives a brief description of what you did and the demonstrable results that were produced

7. Asterisk or dot followed by a descriptive phrase

8. A written summary data sheet or brief account of your qualifications and progress in your chosen career

9. Action words used to describe your attributes and strengths

10. A letter used to introduce yourself and your résumé to a prospective employer with the goal of obtaining an interview

11. Résumé format used when you have employment experience

12. A meeting in which you discuss employment opportunities and strengths that you can bring to the organization

13. Form used to keep track of employment contact information, such as name of employer, name of contact person, address and telephone number, date of first contact, résumé sent, interview date, and follow-up information and dates

LEARNING REVIEW

Short Answer

1. List three types of professionals that would make excellent reference choices.

_____

_____

2. Identify an individual you know personally or have contact with who fits each professional reference type listed above and tell why you think they would be an excellent reference for you.

_____

_____

3. Identify the situations in which using a targeted résumé is advantageous by circling the number next to the statements that apply.

   (1) You are just starting your career and have little experience, but you know what you want and you are clear about your capabilities.

   (2) You want to use one résumé for several different applications.

   (3) You are not clear about your abilities and accomplishments.

   (4) You can go in several directions, and you want a different résumé for each.

   (5) You are able to keep your résumé on a computer disk.

4. Identify the situations in which using a chronological résumé is advantageous by circling the number next to the statements that apply.

   (1) The position is in a highly traditional field.

   (2) Your job history shows real growth and development.

   (3) You are changing career goals.

   (4) You are looking for your first job.

   (5) You are staying in the same field as prior jobs.

5. Identify the situations in which using a functional résumé is advantageous by circling the number next to the statements that apply.

   (1) You have extensive specialized experience.

   (2) Your most recent employers have been highly prestigious.

   (3) You have had a variety of different, apparently unconnected, work experiences.

   (4) You want to emphasize a management growth pattern.

   (5) Much of your work has been volunteer, freelance, or temporary.

6. List four guidelines that are essential when preparing an effective cover letter.

_____

_____

_____

_____

_____

_____

_____

_____

_____

_____

_____

7. List four items that are important when completing a job application.

_____

_____

_____

_____

_____

8. Bob Thompson has an interview at Inner City Health Care for a new clinical medical assisting position. He is confident that he has prepared well for the interview. On the way to the interview, Bob reminds himself of three principles he has learned about interviewing.

(1) _____ before answering questions, and try to provide the information requested in a professional manner.

(2) _____ carefully so that you understand what information the interviewer is requesting.

(3) _____ if you are uncertain.

9. How would you "dress for success" when preparing for your interview?

_____

_____

_____

_____

_____

_____

CERTIFICATION REVIEW

These questions are designed to mimic the certification examination. Select the best response.

1. Telling your friends, family, personal provider, dentist, and ophthalmologist that you are looking for a position in health care is called:

   a. networking

   b. references

   c. professionalism

   d. critiquing

2. Summarizing employment is acceptable on a résumé if it is prior to how many years ago?

   a. 1 year

   b. 5 years

   c. 10 years

   d. 15 years

3. The type of résumé that should be developed by someone who is just starting a career and has little experience is a(n):

   a. targeted résumé

   b. chronological résumé

   c. functional résumé

   d. objective résumé

4. Poise includes such things as:

   a. skill level

   b. confidence and appearance

   c. a. and b.

   d. none of the above

5. Providing a second opportunity to express your interest in an organization and a position may be done with a:

   a. cover letter

   b. recommendation letter

   c. follow-up letter

   d. strategic letter

6. Your attitude is reflected in how you react to:

   a. taking direction

   b. seeking excellence or doing just enough to get by

   c. assuming responsibility for your actions and considering your problems not to be someone else's fault

   d. all of the above

7. Some examples of transferable skills are *(circle all that apply):*

   a. leadership

   b. communication

   c. keyboarding

   d. drawing blood

8. When using someone as a reference, you should:

   a. always ask permission first before the name is printed on the reference list

   b. use your relatives

   c. verify correct spelling, title, place of employment and position, and telephone number

   d. a. and c.

9. Circle the top errors found with résumés.

   a. Typographical and grammatical errors

   b. Not mentioning jobs having transferable skills

   c. Using the same résumé for all job applications

   d. Listing your credentials

10. During the interview, it is *not* appropriate to ask:

    a. if this is a newly created position

    b. if there are opportunities for advancement

    c. about salary, sick leave, benefits, or vacation

    d. what the interviewer considers to be the most difficult task on the job

LEARNING APPLICATION

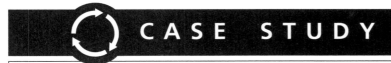
CASE STUDY

CASE STUDY REVIEW QUESTIONS

1. You are the subject of this case study. Complete the Self-Evaluation Worksheet that follows. Use your answers to help you determine the working environment you are most interested in and that best suits you. The worksheet can become a useful tool when researching prospective employers to target for your exciting first job in the medical assisting profession.

SELF-EVALUATION WORKSHEET

Respond to the following questions honestly and sincerely. They are meant to assist you in self-assessment.

1. List your strongest attributes as related to people, data, or things.

   i.e., Interpersonal skills related to people

     Accuracy related to data

     Mechanical ability related to things

   _____ related to _____

   _____ related to _____

   _____ related to _____

2. List your three weakest attributes related to people, data, or things.

   _____ related to _____

   _____ related to _____

   _____ related to _____

3. How do you express yourself? excellent, good, fair, poor

   Orally_____ In writing _____

4. Do you work well as a leader of a group or team? Yes _____ No_____

5. Do you prefer to work alone and on your own? Yes _____ No_____

6. Can you work under stress/pressure? Yes _____ No_____

7. Do you enjoy new ideas and situations? Yes_____ No _____

8. Are you comfortable with routines/schedules? Yes_____ No_____

9. Which work setting do you prefer?

   Single-physician setting _____ Multiphysician setting _____

   Small clinic setting _____ Large clinic setting _____

   Single-specialty setting?_____ Multispecialty setting _____

10. Are you willing to relocate? _____ Willing to travel? _____

Application Activities

1. In the Case Study, you completed a self-assessment form to help you find the type of working environment you are most interested in and best suits you. Create a contact tracker file for yourself, based on the one shown in Figure 25-2 in your textbook. Compile a list from the Yellow Pages, the Internet, want ads in your local paper, your program director, and other sources (hint: other sources are listed in the textbook).

2. Refer to Figure 25-10 in your textbook, which lists typical questions asked during an interview. Write what you would say to a potential employer in response to all of these questions. Then role play with another student, acting as interviewer and interviewee, with these questions and answers to gain confidence for an interview.

3. Recall that the interview process is a "two-way street." You, as the interviewee, should interview the employer. The text lists several example questions you might ask the interviewer during an interview. Develop a list of at least two additional questions that are important to you during the interview process.

CHAPTER POST-TEST

Perform this test without looking at your book. If an answer is "false," rewrite the sentence to make it true.

1. True or False? Positive thinking is a good thing, but it is not all that important to success in planning your career and doing your job search.

_____

_____

2. True or False? When beginning your job search, it would be beneficial to network with students who have graduated before you and are now successfully employed in the field.

_____

_____

3. True or False? Professional appearance is one reason for employers to want to hire a job seeker.

_____

_____

4. True or False? Employers do not expect that you will know it all. They appreciate it when you ask questions.

_____

_____

5. True or False? Students often receive job offers from the office where they extern.

_____

_____

6. True or False? When filling out an application, it is never acceptable to leave answers blank or to write "see résumé."

_____

_____

7. True or False? Plan ahead and have all your information with you when you pick up an application, just in case you are asked to fill it out right there.

_____

_____

SELF-ASSESSMENT

Imagine you are interviewing a recent graduate for a medical assisting position.

1. What questions might you ask during the interviewing process?

_____

_____

_____

_____

2. Do you think you could determine the best person for the job by meeting him or her just once? What else might you do to get to know the person better or get to know his or her work style better?

_____

_____

_____

_____

3. Did the applicant use power verbs effectively? Did they pique your interest?

_____

_____

_____

Competency Assessment Tracking Sheet

Student Name: _____

Procedure Number and Title	Date Assessment Completed and Competency Achieved			
	Date/Initials	**Date/Initials**	**Date/Initials**	**Date/Initials**
EXAMPLE: 22-1 Completing a Medical Incident Report	**2/23/XX DF**	**3/15/XX SL**	**4/20/XX SP**	**5/1/XX JP**
4-1 Identifying Community Resources				
9-1 Control of Bleeding				
9-2 Applying an Arm Splint				
11-1 Booting Up and Shutting Down the Computer				
11-2 Software Installation				
11-3 Hardware Installation				
12-1 Answering and Screening Incoming Calls				
12-2 Transferring a Call				
12-3 Taking a Telephone Message				
12-4 Calling a Pharmacy to Refill an Authorized Prescription				
12-5 Handling Problem Calls				
12-6 Placing Outgoing Calls				
12-7 Recording a Telephone Message on an Answering Device or Voice Mail System				
12-8 Preparing, Sending, and Receiving a Fax				
13-1 Establishing the Appointment Matrix in a Paper System				
13-2 Establishing the Appointment Matrix Using Medical Office Simulation Software (MOSS)				
13-3 Making an Appointment on the Telephone Using Paper Scheduling				
13-4 Making an Appointment on the Telephone Using Medical Office Simulation Software (MOSS)				
13-5 Checking in Patients in a Paper System				

Procedure Number and Title	Date Assessment Completed and Competency Achieved			
	Date/Initials	Date/Initials	Date/Initials	Date/Initials
13-6 Checking in Patients Using Medical Office Simulation Software (MOSS)				
13-7 Cancellation and Rescheduling Procedures Using Paper Scheduling				
13-8 Cancellation and Rescheduling in Medical Office Simulation Software (MOSS)				
13-9 Scheduling Inpatient and Outpatient Admissions and Procedures				
14-1 Establishing a Paper Medical Chart for a New Patient				
14-2 Establishing an Electronic Medical Record for a New Patient Using Medical Office Simulation Software (MOSS)				
14-3 Correcting a Paper Medical Record				
14-4 Correcting an Electronic Medical Record				
14-5 Steps for Manual Filing with an Alphabetic System				
14-6 Steps for Manual Filing with a Numeric System				
14-7 Steps for Manual Filing with a Subject Filing System				
15-1 Preparing and Composing Business Correspondence Using All Components (Computerized Approach)				
15-2 Addressing Envelopes According to United States Postal Regulations				
15-3 Folding Letters for Standard Envelopes				
15-4 Creating a Mass Mailing Using Mail Merge				
15-5 Preparing Outgoing Mail According to United States Postal Regulations				
17-1 Applying Managed Care Policies and Procedures				
17-2 Screening for Insurance				

Procedure Number and Title	Date Assessment Completed and Competency Achieved			
	Date/Initials	Date/Initials	Date/Initials	Date/Initials
17-3 Obtaining Referrals and Authorizations				
17-4 Computing the Medicare Fee Schedule				
18-1 Current Procedural Terminology Coding				
18-2 International Classification of Diseases, 9th Revision, Clinical Modification Coding				
18-3 Applying Third-Party Guidelines				
18-4 Completing a Medicare CMS-1500 (08-05) Claim Form				
19-1 Recording/Posting Patient Charges, Payments, and Adjustments in a Manual System				
19-2 Balancing Day Sheets in a Manual System				
19-3 Posting Patient Charges Using Medical Office Simulation Software (MOSS)				
19-4 Insurance Billing Using Medical Office Simulation Software (MOSS)				
19-5 Posting Payments and Adjustments Using Medical Office Simulation Software (MOSS)				
19-6 Processing Credit Balances and Refunds Using Medical Office Simulation Software (MOSS)				
19-7 Preparing a Deposit				
19-8 Recording a Nonsufficient Funds Check in a Manual System				
19-9 Writing a Check				
19-10 Reconciling a Bank Statement				
19-11 Establishing and Maintaining a Petty Cash Fund				
20-1 Explaining Fees in the First Telephone Interview				
20-2 Prepare Itemized Patient Accounts for Billing in a Manual System				

Procedure Number and Title	Date Assessment Completed and Competency Achieved			
	Date/Initials	**Date/Initials**	**Date/Initials**	**Date/Initials**
20-3 Identify Accounts Receivable Using Medical Office Simulation Software (MOSS)				
20-4 Preparing Itemized Patient Accounts for Billing Using Medical Office Simulation Software (MOSS)				
20-5 Post/Record Collection Agency Adjustments in a Manual System				
20-6 Post/Record Adjustments Using Medical Office Simulation Software (MOSS)				
21-1 Preparing Accounts Receivable Trial Balance in a Manual System				
21-2 Preparing Accounts Receivable Trial Balance Using Medical Office Simulation Software (MOSS)				
22-1 Completing a Medical Incident Report				
22-2 Preparing a Meeting Agenda				
22-3 Supervising a Student Practicum				
22-4 Developing and Maintaining a Procedure Manual				
22-5 Making Travel Arrangements with a Travel Agent				
22-6 Making Travel Arrangements via the Internet				
22-7 Processing Employee Payroll				
22-8 Perform an Inventory of Equipment and Supplies				
22-9 Perform Routine Maintenance or Calibration of Administrative and Clinical Equipment				
23-1 Develop and Maintain a Policy Manual				
23-2 Prepare a Job Description				
23-3 Conduct Interviews				
23-4 Orient Personnel				

Competency
Assessment
Checklists

Name _____   **Date** _____   **Score** _____

COMPETENCY ASSESSMENT

Procedure 4-1   Identifying Community Resources

Task: To have a list of community resources available for patient use.

Conditions: Computer and printer, multiple resources from a variety of community services

Standards: Perform the Task within 30 minutes with a minimum score of _____ points.

Work
Documentation: Electronic database or notebook of resources found

No.	Step	Points	Check #1	Check #2	Check #3
1	Determine the type of information to be in your database.				
2	Contact the sources and request any listings they may have.				
3	Search the Internet to obtain the desired resources.				
4	Develop a database on your computer so you can search easily for the resource when needed. Maintain a notebook with the resource information printed and indexed.				
	Student's Total Points				
	Points Possible				
	Final Score (Student's Total Points/ Possible Points)				

Name _____ **Date** _____ **Score** _____

WORK DOCUMENTATION
*Attach list of resources found.

_____

Instructor's/Evaluator's Comments and Suggestions:

_____
_____
_____
_____
_____

CHECK #1	
Evaluator's Signature:	Date:

CHECK #2	
Evaluator's Signature:	Date:

CHECK #3	
Evaluator's Signature:	Date:

ABHES Competency: VI.A.1.a.3.e Locate resources and information for patients and employers

CAAHEP Curriculum: IV.P.12 Develop and maintain a current list of community resources related to patients' healthcare needs; XI.P.12 Maintain a current list of community resources for emergency preparedness.

Name _____   **Date** _____   **Score** _____

COMPETENCY ASSESSMENT

Procedure 9-1   Control of Bleeding

Task: To control bleeding caused by an open wound.

Conditions: Sterile dressings, sterile gloves, mask, eye protection, a gown, biohazard waste container

Standards: Perform the Task within 15 minutes with a minimum score of _____ points.

Work
Documentation: Simulated entry in Patient's Chart in Work Documentation area

No.	Step	Points	Check #1	Check #2	Check #3
1	Wash hands and gather equipment quickly.				
2	Apply gloves and other PPE; eye mask, gown if splashing likely.				
3	Apply pressure bandages and apply pressure for 10 minutes. If bleeding continues, elevate arm above heart. If continues, press adjacent artery against bone.				
4	Throughout procedure, demonstrate professional behavior in manner, organization and attire, including: • Recognize the effects of stress on all persons involved in emergency situations. • Demonstrate self-awareness in responding to emergency situations.				
5	Dispose of waste in biohazard container and wash hands.				
6	Document procedure.				
Student's Total Points					
Points Possible					
Final Score (Student's Total Points/ Possible Points)					

Name _____ **Date** _____ **Score** _____

WORK DOCUMENTATION

_____

Instructor's/Evaluator's Comments and Suggestions:

_____

_____

_____

_____

_____

CHECK #1	
Evaluator's Signature:	Date:

CHECK #2	
Evaluator's Signature:	Date:

CHECK #3	
Evaluator's Signature:	Date:

ABHES Competency: VI.A.1.a(4)(f) Perform first aid and CPR; VI.A.1.a.4.e Recognize emergencies

CAAHEP Curriculum: XI.P.XI.11 Perform first aid procedures

Name _____   **Date** _____   **Score** _____

COMPETENCY ASSESSMENT

Procedure 9-2   Applying an Arm Splint

Task: To immobilize the area above and below the injured part of the arm to reduce pain and prevent further injury.

Conditions: Thin piece of rigid board and gauze roller bandage

Standards: Perform the Task within 15 minutes with a minimum score of _____ points.

Work
Documentation: Simulated entry in Patient's Chart in Work Documentation area

No.	Step	Points	Check #1	Check #2	Check #3
1	Place a padded splint under the injured area. Hold the splint in place with roller gauze.				
2	Check circulation (note color and temperature of skin and nails, and check pulse).				
3	Apply sling to keep arm elevated.				
4	Throughout procedure, demonstrate professional behavior in manner, organization, and attire, including: • Recognize the effects of stress on all persons involved in emergency situations. • Demonstrate self awareness in responding to emergency situations.				
5	Wash hands.				
6	Document procedure.				
Student's Total Points					
Points Possible					
Final Score (Student's Total Points/ Possible Points)					

Name _____   **Date** _____   **Score** _____

WORK DOCUMENTATION

_____

Instructor's/Evaluator's Comments and Suggestions:

_____
_____
_____
_____
_____

CHECK #1

Evaluator's Signature: Date:

CHECK #2

Evaluator's Signature: Date:

CHECK #3

Evaluator's Signature: Date:

ABHES Competency: VI.A.1.a(4)(f) Perform first aid and CPR

CAAHEP Curriculum: XI.P.XI.11 Perform first aid procedures

Name _____ **Date** _____ **Score** _____

COMPETENCY ASSESSMENT

Procedure 11-1   Booting Up and Shutting Down the Computer

Task: To properly turn on and shut down the computer.

Conditions: Computer, portable media device (such as a flash drive or CD)

Standards: Perform the Task within 10 minutes with a minimum score of _____ points.

No.	Step	Points	Check #1	Check #2	Check #3
1	Turn on the computer and monitor. Log in using a username and password, if applicable.				
2	When work has been completed, save all open files and close all open software programs.				
3	Remove and store all portable media devices (CD, flash drive, etc.) appropriately.				
4	Close out of the operating system, shut down the computer, and power the computer and monitor off.				
Student's Total Points					
Points Possible					
Final Score (Student's Total Points/ Possible Points)					

Name _____   **Date** _____   **Score** _____

Instructor's/Evaluator's Comments and Suggestions:

_____

_____

_____

_____

_____

CHECK #1

Evaluator's Signature: _____   Date:

CHECK #2

Evaluator's Signature: _____   Date:

CHECK #3

Evaluator's Signature: _____   Date:

ABHES Competency: VI.A.1.a.2.n Application of electronic technology

Name _____ **Date** _____ **Score** _____

COMPETENCY ASSESSMENT

Procedure 11-2 Software Installation

Task: To add software to the computer system for later call up and use.

Conditions: Computer, StudyWARE Software CD in back of the textbook (*Note:* students may install any software program as directed by the instructor)

Standards: Perform the Task within 10 minutes with a minimum score of _____ points.

No.	Step	Points	Check #1	Check #2	Check #3
Automatic Installation					
1	Close all open programs.				
2	Insert the CD into the CD drive.				
3	Follow the prompts in the Installation Wizard screens that appear, choosing an appropriate location for the program.				
4	Click Finish and launch the StudyWARE program.				
Manual Installation					
1	Close all open programs.				
2	Insert CD into the CD drive.				
3	From My Computer, double click the icon for the CD drive. Follow the prompts in the Installation Wizard screens that appear, choosing an appropriate location for the program.				
4	Click Finish and launch the StudyWARE program.				
Student's Total Points					
Points Possible					
Final Score (Student's Total Points/ Possible Points)					

Name _____   **Date** _____   **Score** _____

Instructor's/Evaluator's Comments and Suggestions:

_____

_____

_____

_____

_____

CHECK #1

Evaluator's Signature: _____   Date: _____

CHECK #2

Evaluator's Signature: _____   Date: _____

CHECK #3

Evaluator's Signature: _____   Date: _____

ABHES Competency: VI.A.1.a.2.n Application of electronic technology; VI.A.1.a.3.d Apply computer concepts for office procedures

CAAHEP Curriculum: V.P.6 Use office hardware and software to maintain office systems

Name _____   **Date** _____   **Score** _____

COMPETENCY ASSESSMENT

Procedure 11-3   Hardware Installation

Task: To add hardware to the computer system for later use.

Conditions: Computer, hardware to be installed

Standards: Perform the Task within 15 minutes with a minimum score of _____ points.

No.	Step	Points	Check #1	Check #2	Check #3
Using Automatic Initiation from Microsoft Windows® Installation Wizard					
1	Close all open programs.				
2	Answer questions appropriately such as: Manufacturer, Model Number, etc.				
3	Follow onscreen directions.				
Using Manual Initiation of Microsoft Windows® Installation Wizard					
1	Close all open programs.				
2	Go to START, SETTINGS, CONTROL PANEL, and double click ADD HARDWARE.				
3	Find the Hardware you wish to install and follow onscreen instructions.				
Student's Total Points					
Points Possible					
Final Score (Student's Total Points/ Possible Points)					

Name _____ **Date** _____ **Score** _____

Instructor's/Evaluator's Comments and Suggestions:

_____

_____

_____

_____

_____

CHECK #1

Evaluator's Signature: _____ Date:

CHECK #2

Evaluator's Signature: _____ Date:

CHECK #3

Evaluator's Signature: _____ Date:

ABHES Competency: VI.A.1.a.2.n Application of electronic technology; VI.A.1.a.3.d Apply computer concepts for office procedures

CAAHEP Curriculum: V.P.6 Use office hardware and software to maintain office systems

Name _____   **Date** _____   **Score** _____

COMPETENCY ASSESSMENT

Procedure 12-1   Answering and Screening Incoming Calls

Task: To answer telephone calls professionally, acquiring all necessary information from the caller, documenting it correctly, and properly acting on it.

Condition: Telephone, appointment calendar, message pad, pen or pencil, notepad, assessment protocols, Scenario information

Standards: Perform the Task within 15 minutes with a minimum score of _____ points.

Work Documentation: Simulated entry in Patient's Chart in Work Documentation section

No.	Step	Points	Check #1	Check #2	Check #3
1	Answer phone professionally and appropriately. Ask for caller's name and determine if call is an emergency.				
2	Follow established office protocol for screening. Repeat information back to the patient.				
3	During call, demonstrate professional behavior, including: • Demonstrate empathy in communicating with patients, family, and staff • Apply active listening skills • Analyze communications in providing appropriate responses/feedback				
4	End call professionally and appropriately.				
5	Document information and record future necessary actions.				
Student's Total Points					
Points Possible					
Final Score (Student's Total Points/ Possible Points)					

Name _____ **Date** _____ **Score** _____

WORK DOCUMENTATION

_____

Instructor's/Evaluator's Comments and Suggestions:

_____

_____

_____

_____

_____

CHECK #1

Evaluator's Signature: _____ Date: _____

CHECK #2

Evaluator's Signature: _____ Date: _____

CHECK #3

Evaluator's Signature: _____ Date: _____

ABHES Competency: VI.A.1.a.2.e Use proper telephone techniques; VI.A.1.a.2.h Receive, organize, prioritize, and transmit information expediently

CAAHEP Curriculum: IV.P.7 Demonstrate telephone techniques; IV.P.2 Report relevant information to others succinctly and accurately

Name _____ **Date** _____ **Score** _____

COMPETENCY ASSESSMENT

Procedure 12-2 Transferring a Call

Task: To transfer a call directly to the individual who can handle the call in an efficient and professional manner.

Condition: Telephone, message pad, black ink pen, notepad, interoffice telephone directory, Scenario information

Standards: Perform the Task within 3 minutes with a minimum score of _____ points.

No.	Step	Points	Check #1	Check #2	Check #3
1	Answer call professionally and appropriately.				
2	Obtain the name and phone number of individual, and write down notes regarding situation.				
3	During call, demonstrate professional behavior, including: • Demonstrate empathy in communicating with patients, family, and staff • Apply active listening skills • Analyze communications in providing appropriate responses/feedback				
4	Ask caller for permission before placing him or her on hold.				
5	Determine the best individual to take the call and transfer the call.				
Student's Total Points					
Points Possible					
Final Score (Student's Total Points/ Possible Points)					

Name _____   **Date** _____   **Score** _____

Instructor's/Evaluator's Comments and Suggestions:

_____

_____

_____

_____

_____

CHECK #1

Evaluator's Signature: _____   Date: _____

CHECK #2

Evaluator's Signature: _____   Date: _____

CHECK #3

Evaluator's Signature: _____   Date: _____

ABHES Competency: VI.A.1.a.2.e Use proper telephone techniques; VI.A.1.a.2.h Receive, organize, prioritize, and transmit information expediently

CAAHEP Curriculum: IV.P.7 Demonstrate telephone techniques

Name _____ **Date** _____ **Score** _____

COMPETENCY ASSESSMENT

Procedure 12-3   Taking a Telephone Message

Task: To record an accurate message and follow up as required.

Condition: Telephone, message pad, black ink pen, notepad, clock or watch, Scenario information

Standards: Perform the Task within 5 minutes with a minimum score of _____ points.

Work Documentation: Simulated phone message in Work Documentation section or message form

No.	Step	Points	Check #1	Check #2	Check #3
1	Answer the call professionally and appropriately.				
2	Gather all appropriate information from caller on a message pad; repeat information back to caller.				
3	During call, demonstrate professional behavior, including: • Demonstrate empathy in communicating with patients, family, and staff • Apply active listening skills • Demonstrate sensitivity to the message being delivered • Analyze communications in providing appropriate responses/feedback				
4	End call professionally and appropriately.				
5	Document the phone message in the patient's medical record.				
6	Deliver message to the intended individual.				
Student's Total Points					
Points Possible					
Final Score (Student's Total Points/ Possible Points)					

Name _____   **Date** _____   **Score** _____

WORK DOCUMENTATION

_____

Instructor's/Evaluator's Comments and Suggestions:

_____

_____

_____

_____

CHECK #1

Evaluator's Signature: _____   Date:

CHECK #2

Evaluator's Signature: _____   Date:

CHECK #3

Evaluator's Signature: _____   Date:

ABHES Competency: VI.A.1.a.2.e Use proper telephone techniques; VI.A.1.a.2.h Receive, organize, prioritize, and transmit information expediently; VI.A.1.a.5.b Document accurately

CAAHEP Curriculum: IV.P.7 Demonstrate telephone techniques; IV.P.2 Report relevant information to others succinctly and accurately; IV.P.8 Document patient care

Name _____ **Date** _____ **Score** _____

COMPETENCY ASSESSMENT

Procedure 12-4   Calling a Pharmacy to Refill an Authorized Prescription

Task: To notify a pharmacy to refill an authorized prescription.

Condition: Patient's chart, message pad, pen, Scenario information

Standards: Perform the Task within 15 minutes with a minimum score of _____ points.

Work Documentation: Simulated entry in Patient's Chart in Work Documentation section

No.	Step	Points	Check #1	Check #2	Check #3
1	Receive patient's call and obtain appropriate information from patient.				
2	During call, demonstrate professional behavior, including: • Demonstrate empathy in communicating with patients, family, and staff • Apply active listening skills • Analyze communications in providing appropriate responses/feedback				
3	Attach the completed message to patient's chart and give to the provider.				
4	If the refill is approved by the provider, call the pharmacy with appropriate refill information.				
5	Document the call accurately in the patient's chart.				
Student's Total Points					
Points Possible					
Final Score (Student's Total Points/ Possible Points)					

Name _____   **Date** _____   **Score** _____

WORK DOCUMENTATION

_____

Instructor's/Evaluator's Comments and Suggestions:

_____
_____
_____
_____
_____

CHECK #1

Evaluator's Signature: Date:

CHECK #2

Evaluator's Signature: Date:

CHECK #3

Evaluator's Signature: Date:

ABHES Competency: VI.A.1.a.2.d Serve as liaison between Physician and others; VI.A.1.a.2.e Use proper telephone techniques; VI.A.1.a.5.b Document accurately

CAAHEP Curriculum: IV.P.7 Demonstrate telephone techniques; IV.P.8 Document patient care

Name _____   **Date** _____   **Score** _____

COMPETENCY ASSESSMENT

Procedure 12-5   Handling Problem Calls

Task: To handle calls in a positive and professional manner while providing necessary comfort, empathy, and information to the caller to resolve the problem.

Condition: Telephone, message pad, pen or pencil, Scenario information

Standards: Perform the Task within 15 minutes with a minimum score of _____ points.

Work
Documentation: Simulated entry in Patient's Chart in Work Documentation section

No.	Step	Points	Check #1	Check #2	Check #3
1	Answer the phone professionally and appropriately. Remain calm and avoid becoming upset.				
2	Listen to what the caller is upset about, then paraphrase back to the caller for verification.				
3	If the call is an emergency, begin screening procedures as needed. Finalize and follow through on action to be taken.				
4	During call, demonstrate professional behavior, including: • Demonstrate empathy in communicating with patients, family, and staff • Apply active listening skills • Demonstrate sensitivity to the message being delivered • Analyze communications in providing appropriate responses/feedback				
5	End call professionally and appropriately.				
6	Document the call accurately.				
7	Report the call to the office manager.				
Student's Total Points					
Points Possible					
Final Score (Student's Total Points/ Possible Points)					

Name _____   **Date** _____   **Score** _____

WORK DOCUMENTATION

Instructor's/Evaluator's Comments and Suggestions:

_____

_____

_____

_____

_____

CHECK #1

Evaluator's Signature: _____   Date:

CHECK #2

Evaluator's Signature: _____   Date:

CHECK #3

Evaluator's Signature: _____   Date:

ABHES Competency: VI.A.1.a.2.e Use proper telephone techniques; VI.A.1.a.2.h Receive, organize, prioritize, and transmit information expediently; VI.A.1.a.5.b Document accurately

CAAHEP Curriculum: IV.P.7 Demonstrate telephone techniques; IV.P.2 Report relevant information to others succinctly and accurately; IV.P.8 Document patient care

Name _____   **Date** _____   **Score** _____

COMPETENCY ASSESSMENT

Procedure 12-6   Placing Outgoing Calls

Task: To place calls efficiently and effectively.

Condition: Telephone, notepad, pen or pencil, all materials specifically applicable to the call

Standards: Perform the Task within 3 minutes with a minimum score of _____ points.

Work
Documentation: Simulated entry in Patient's Chart in Work Documentation section

No.	Step	Points	Check #1	Check #2	Check #3
1	Prepare all materials to make the call.				
2	Use appropriate language and tone, and follow proper telephone techniques.				
3	Complete calls correctly and professionally for the specific situation.				
4	During call, demonstrate professional behavior, including: • Demonstrate empathy in communicating with patients, family, and staff • Apply active listening skills • Demonstrate recognition of the patient's level of understanding in communications • Analyze communications in providing appropriate responses/feedback				
5	Document appropriately.				
Student's Total Points					
Points Possible					
Final Score (Student's Total Points/ Possible Points)					

Name _____ **Date** _____ **Score** _____

WORK DOCUMENTATION

_____

Instructor's/Evaluator's Comments and Suggestions:

_____

_____

_____

_____

_____

CHECK #1

Evaluator's Signature: _____ Date: _____

CHECK #2

Evaluator's Signature: _____ Date: _____

CHECK #3

Evaluator's Signature: _____ Date: _____

ABHES Competency: VI.A.1.a.2.e Use proper telephone techniques; VI.A.1.a.2.h Receive, organize, prioritize, and transmit information expediently; VI.A.1.a.5.b Document accurately

CAAHEP Curriculum: IV.P.7 Demonstrate telephone techniques; IV.P.2 Report relevant information to others succinctly and accurately; IV.P.8 Document patient care

Name _____ **Date** _____ **Score** _____

COMPETENCY ASSESSMENT

Procedure 12-7   Recording a Telephone Message on an Answering Device or Voice Mail System

Task: To provide clear and precise instructions to the caller when medical staff is not available to answer the call immediately.

Condition: Telephone and recording device, prepared written message to record

Standards: Perform the Task within 15 minutes with a minimum score of _____ points.

No.	Step	Points	Check #1	Check #2	Check #3
1	Write out message to be recorded, then record the message on the device.				
2	Play the message back to verify that it is accurate and includes all necessary information.				
3	Set the message device to the recorded message when you are not available to answer.				
Student's Total Points					
Points Possible					
Final Score (Student's Total Points/ Possible Points)					

Name _____   **Date** _____   **Score** _____

Instructor's/Evaluator's Comments and Suggestions:

_____

_____

_____

_____

_____

CHECK #1

Evaluator's Signature: _____   Date: _____

CHECK #2

Evaluator's Signature: _____   Date: _____

CHECK #3

Evaluator's Signature: _____   Date: _____

ABHES Competency: VI.A.1.a.2.e Use proper telephone techniques; VI.A.1.a.3.a Perform basic secretarial skills

CAAHEP Curriculum: IV.P.7 Demonstrate telephone techniques

Name _____ **Date** _____ **Score** _____

COMPETENCY ASSESSMENT

Procedure 12-8   Preparing, Sending, and Receiving a Fax

Task: To send and receive information quickly and accurately by fax (facsimile).

Condition: Fax machine, telephone

Standards: Perform the Task within 15 minutes with a minimum score of _____ points.

Work
Documentation: Completed fax cover sheet

No.	Step	Points	Check #1	Check #2	Check #3
1	Prepare a cover sheet.				
2	Turn on fax machine. Place the document according to machine instructions, and dial the fax number of the receiver.				
3	After document passes through, press button requesting a receipt. Remove the document and call recipient to verify delivery.				
4	To receive: Turn on fax machine, and check to see that phone line is available.				
5	Remove document from machine after it is received and deliver to addressee.				
Student's Total Points					
Points Possible					
Final Score (Student's Total Points/ Possible Points)					

Name _____   **Date** _____   **Score** _____

WORK DOCUMENTATION

*Attach printed fax cover sheet.

Instructor's/Evaluator's Comments and Suggestions:

_____

_____

_____

_____

_____

CHECK #1	
Evaluator's Signature:	Date:

CHECK #2	
Evaluator's Signature:	Date:

CHECK #3	
Evaluator's Signature:	Date:

ABHES Competency: VI.A.1.a.2.h Receive, organize, prioritize, and transmit information expediently; VI.A.1.a.3.a Perform basic secretarial skills

CAAHEP Curriculum: IV.P.2 Report relevant information to others succinctly and accurately

Name _____   **Date** _____   **Score** _____

COMPETENCY ASSESSMENT

Procedure 13-1   Establishing the Appointment Matrix in a Paper System

Task: To have a current and accurate record of appointment times available for scheduling patient visits, in a paper system.

Condition: Appointment scheduler, clinic schedule, provider and staff schedule, office calendar

Standards: Perform the Task within 15 minutes with a minimum score of _____ points.

Work Documentation: Completed appointment matrix

No.	Step	Points	Check #1	Check #2	Check #3
1	Mark in appointment book times that are not to be scheduled; indicate all vacations, holidays, and other office closures.				
2	Correctly block off times for all provider meetings, hospital rounds, appointments, conferences, vacations, and other prescheduled commitments.				
	Student's Total Points				
	Points Possible				
	Final Score (Student's Total Points/ Possible Points)				

Name _____   **Date** _____   **Score** _____

WORK DOCUMENTATION
*Attach completed appointment matrix.

_____

Instructor's/Evaluator's Comments and Suggestions:

_____
_____
_____
_____
_____

CHECK #1

Evaluator's Signature: _____   Date:

CHECK #2

Evaluator's Signature: _____   Date:

CHECK #3

Evaluator's Signature: _____   Date:

ABHES Competency: VI.A.1.a.3.c Schedule and monitor appointments

CAAHEP Curriculum: V.P.1 Manage appointment schedule, using established priorities

Name _____ Date _____ Score _____

COMPETENCY ASSESSMENT

Procedure 13-2   Establishing the Appointment Matrix Using Medical Office Simulation Software (MOSS)

Task: To have a current and accurate record of appointment times available for scheduling patient visits, in an electronic system.

Condition: MOSS, computer, Scenario information

Standards: Perform the Task within 15 minutes with a minimum score of _____ points.

Work Documentation: Screen shots of completed block calendar window or screen shots of the appointment schedule showing calendar blocks

No.	Step	Points	Check #1	Check #2	Check #3
1	Open MOSS, select the Appointment Scheduling module.				
2	Find the appropriate date; select Block Calendar option.				
3	Enter correct information for the type of block, the start and end dates, the start and end times, the frequency, and the providers to whom the blocks apply. (Take screen shots of the complete block calendar window.)				
4	Save each calendar block, and review the schedule to ensure that each block has been properly applied. (Take screen shots of the appointment schedule showing the calendar blocks.)				
Student's Total Points					
Points Possible					
Final Score (Student's Total Points/ Possible Points)					

Name _____   **Date** _____   **Score** _____

WORK DOCUMENTATION

*Attach screen shots of completed block calendar window or screen shots of the appointment schedule showing calendar blocks.

Instructor's/Evaluator's Comments and Suggestions:

_____
_____
_____
_____
_____

CHECK #1

Evaluator's Signature: _____   Date: _____

CHECK #2

Evaluator's Signature: _____   Date: _____

CHECK #3

Evaluator's Signature: _____   Date: _____

ABHES Competency: VI.A.1.a.2.n Application of electronic technology; VI.A.1.a.3.c Schedule and monitor appointments; VI.A.1.a.3.d Apply computer concepts for office procedures

CAAHEP Curriculum: V.P.1 Manage appointment schedule, using established priorities; V.P.6 Use office hardware and software to maintain office systems

Name _____ **Date** _____ **Score** _____

COMPETENCY ASSESSMENT

Procedure 13-3 Making an Appointment on the Telephone Using Paper Scheduling

Task: To schedule an appointment entering information in the appointment schedule according to office policy.

Condition: Telephone, black ink pen, calendar, appointment matrix

Standards: Perform the Task within 15 minutes with a minimum score of _____ points.

Work Documentation: Appointment matrix with completed patient entry

No.	Step	Points	Check #1	Check #2	Check #3
1	Answer phone professionally and appropriately.				
2	Make notes on your personal log sheet of patient's name and reason for calling. Determine if patient is new or established, provider to be seen, and reason for appointment; search for an available time that is convenient for the patient.				
3	During call, demonstrate professional behavior, including: • Demonstrate empathy in communicating with patients, family, and staff • Apply active listening skills • Demonstrate recognition of the patient's level of understanding in communications • Analyze communications in providing appropriate responses/feedback				
4	Correctly enter patient's name into the schedule; repeat the date and time to the patient, and provide any necessary instructions; end the call politely.				
5	Recheck your personal log sheet and ensure all information was transferred into the schedule. Draw a line through the notes, when finished.				
Student's Total Points					
Points Possible					
Final Score (Student's Total Points/ Possible Points)					

Name _____   **Date** _____   **Score** _____

WORK DOCUMENTATION
*Attach completed appointment matrix.

_____

Instructor's/Evaluator's Comments and Suggestions:

_____

_____

_____

_____

_____

CHECK #1

Evaluator's Signature: _____   Date:

CHECK #2

Evaluator's Signature: _____   Date:

CHECK #3

Evaluator's Signature: _____   Date:

ABHES Competency: VI.A.1.a.2.e Use proper telephone techniques; VI.A.1.a.3.c Schedule and monitor appointments

CAAHEP Curriculum: IV.P.7 Demonstrate telephone techniques; V.P.1 Manage appointment schedule, using established priorities

Name _____   **Date** _____   **Score** _____

COMPETENCY ASSESSMENT

Procedure 13-4   Making an Appointment on the Telephone Using Medical Office Simulation Software (MOSS)

Task: To schedule an appointment entering information in the appointment schedule according to office policy.

Condition: Telephone, MOSS, computer, Scenario information

Standards: Perform the Task within 15 minutes with a minimum score of _____ points.

Work Documentation: Screen shot of the completed Patient Appointment Form

No.	Step	Points	Check #1	Check #2	Check #3
1	Answer phone professionally and appropriately.				
2	Open MOSS, select the Appointment Scheduling module. Find and select the appropriate date for the appointment, and the appropriate patient.				
3	During call, demonstrate professional behavior, including: • Demonstrate empathy in communicating with patients, family, and staff • Apply active listening skills • Demonstrate recognition of the patient's level of understanding in communications • Analyze communications in providing appropriate responses/feedback				
4	Populate the fields on the Patient Appointment Form with the correct information. (Take a screen shot of the completed Patient Appointment Form.)				
5	Save the appointment, and review the schedule to ensure that the appointment was properly applied.				
6	Repeat the date and time to the patient, provide any necessary instructions; end the call politely.				
	Student's Total Points				
	Points Possible				
	Final Score (Student's Total Points/ Possible Points)				

Name _____ Date _____ Score _____

WORK DOCUMENTATION

*Attach screen shot of completed Patient Appointment Form.

Instructor's/Evaluator's Comments and Suggestions:

_____

_____

_____

_____

_____

CHECK #1

Evaluator's Signature: _____ Date:

CHECK #2

Evaluator's Signature: _____ Date:

CHECK #3

Evaluator's Signature: _____ Date:

ABHES Competency: VI.A.1.a.2.e Use proper telephone techniques; VI.A.1.a.2.n Application of electronic technology; VI.A.1.a.3.c Schedule and monitor appointments; VI.A.1.a.3.d Apply computer concepts for office procedures

CAAHEP Curriculum: IV.P.7 Demonstrate telephone techniques; V.P.1 Manage appointment schedule, using established priorities; V.P.6 Use office hardware and software to maintain office systems

Name _____ **Date** _____ **Score** _____

COMPETENCY ASSESSMENT

Procedure 13-5   Checking in Patients in a Paper System

Task: To ensure the patient is given prompt and proper care; to meet legal safeguards for documentation.

Condition: Patient chart, black ink pen, required forms, check-in list, appointment book, Scenario information

Standards: Perform the Task within 25 minutes with a minimum score of _____ points.

Work Documentation: Completed appointment book page

No.	Step	Points	Check #1	Check #2	Check #3
1	Prepare a list of patients to be seen and assemble the charts; check charts to see that everything is up to date.				
2	Acknowledge patients when they arrive.				
3	Indicate patient's arrival on daily worksheet. Ask patient to be seated and indicate wait time.				
4	During exchange with patient: • Review vital information, protect patient privacy • Recognize and protect personal boundaries in communicating with others				
5	Following office policy, place the chart where it can be picked up to route the patient to the appropriate location for the visit.				
Student's Total Points					
Points Possible					
Final Score (Student's Total Points/ Possible Points)					

Name _____ **Date** _____ **Score** _____

WORK DOCUMENTATION

*Attach completed appointment book page.

Instructor's/Evaluator's Comments and Suggestions:

_____
_____
_____
_____
_____

CHECK #1

Evaluator's Signature: Date:

CHECK #2

Evaluator's Signature: Date:

CHECK #3

Evaluator's Signature: Date:

ABHES Competency: VI.A.1.a.3.c Schedule and monitor appointments

CAAHEP Curriculum: IV.P.2 Report relevant information to others succinctly and accurately; V.P.1 Manage appointment schedule, using established priorities

Name _____   **Date** _____   **Score** _____

COMPETENCY ASSESSMENT

Procedure 13-6   Checking in Patients Using Medical Office Simulation Software (MOSS)

Task: To ensure the patient is given prompt and proper care; to meet legal safeguards for documentation.

Condition: MOSS, computer, Scenario information

Standards: Perform the Task within 5 minutes with a minimum score of _____ points.

Work Documentation: Screen shot of completed Patient Appointment Form

No.	Step	Points	Check #1	Check #2	Check #3
1	Open MOSS, select the Appointment Scheduling module. Find and select the appropriate date for the appointment, and the appropriate patient.				
2	Check in the patient on the Patient Appointment Form with the correct information in the correct field. (Take a screen shot of the completed Patient Appointment Form.)				
3	During exchange with patient: • Review vital information, protect privacy • Recognize and protect personal boundaries in communicating with others				
4	Save the appointment. Ask patient to be seated and indicate wait time.				
Student's Total Points					
Points Possible					
Final Score (Student's Total Points/ Possible Points)					

Name _____   **Date** _____   **Score** _____

WORK DOCUMENTATION

*Attach screen shot of completed Patient Appointment Form.

_____

Instructor's/Evaluator's Comments and Suggestions:

_____

_____

_____

_____

_____

CHECK #1	
Evaluator's Signature:	Date:

CHECK #2	
Evaluator's Signature:	Date:

CHECK #3	
Evaluator's Signature:	Date:

ABHES Competency: VI.A.1.a.3.c Schedule and monitor appointments

CAAHEP Curriculum: IV.P.2 Report relevant information to others succinctly and accurately; V.P.1 Manage appointment schedule, using established priorities

Name _____ **Date** _____ **Score** _____

COMPETENCY ASSESSMENT

Procedure 13-7   Cancellation and Rescheduling Procedures Using Paper Scheduling

Task: To protect the provider from legal complications; to free up care time for other patients; and to assure quality patient care.

Condition: Patient chart, red ink pen, check-in list, appointment book, Scenario information

Standards: Perform the Task within 15 minutes with a minimum score of _____ points.

Work Documentation: Appointment schedule with change indication; documentation in patient's chart

No.	Step	Points	Check #1	Check #2	Check #3
1	Indicate on the appointment sheet all appointments that were changed, canceled, or did not show.				
2	Reschedule those appointments by calling the patients. If unable to reschedule, record a reminder in the tickler file.				
3	During interaction with patient, demonstrate professional behavior, including: • Demonstrate empathy in communicating with patients, family, and staff • Apply active listening skills • Demonstrate recognition of the patient's level of understanding in communications • Analyze communications in providing appropriate responses/feedback				
4	Document action taken in the patient's chart.				
Student's Total Points					
Points Possible					
Final Score (Student's Total Points/ Possible Points)					

Name _____   **Date** _____   **Score** _____

WORK DOCUMENTATION
*Attach appointment schedule.

Instructor's/Evaluator's Comments and Suggestions:

_____

_____

_____

_____

_____

CHECK #1

Evaluator's Signature: _____   Date:

CHECK #2

Evaluator's Signature: _____   Date:

CHECK #3

Evaluator's Signature: _____   Date:

ABHES Competency: VI.A.1.a.3.c Schedule and monitor appointments

CAAHEP Curriculum: IV.P.8 Document patient care; V.P.1 Manage appointment schedule, using established priorities

Name _____ Date _____ Score _____

COMPETENCY ASSESSMENT

Procedure 13-8   Cancellation and Rescheduling in Medical Office
Simulation Software (MOSS)

Task: To protect the provider from legal complications; to free up care time for other patients; and to assure quality patient care.

Condition: MOSS, computer, Scenario information

Standards: Perform the Task within 15 minutes with a minimum score of _____ points.

Work Documentation: Screen shot of Patient Appointment Form

No.	Step	Points	Check #1	Check #2	Check #3
1	Open MOSS, select the Appointment Scheduling module. Using the Scenario information, find and select the appropriate date, and the appropriate patient.				
2	*Rescheduling:* Choose "Rescheduled" on the Patient Appointment Form, select the reason and find a new time to reschedule the patient. (Take a screen shot of the completed Patient Appointment Form.) *Cancellations:* Choose "Cancelled," select the reason. (Take a screen shot of the completed Patient Appointment Form.)				
3	During interaction with patient, demonstrate professional behavior, including: • Demonstrate empathy in communicating with patients, family, and staff • Apply active listening skills • Demonstrate recognition of the patient's level of understanding in communications • Analyze communications in providing appropriate responses/feedback				
4	Save the appointment changes.				
Student's Total Points					
Points Possible					
Final Score (Student's Total Points/ Possible Points)					

Name _____ **Date** _____ **Score** _____

WORK DOCUMENTATION

*Attach screen shot of completed Patient Appointment Form.

_____

Instructor's/Evaluator's Comments and Suggestions:

_____

_____

_____

_____

_____

CHECK #1

Evaluator's Signature: _____   Date: _____

CHECK #2

Evaluator's Signature: _____   Date: _____

CHECK #3

Evaluator's Signature: _____   Date: _____

ABHES Competency: VI.A.1.a.2.n Application of electronic technology; VI.A.1.a.3.c Schedule and monitor appointments; VI.A.1.a.3.d Apply computer concepts for office procedures

CAAHEP Curriculum: IV.P.8 Document patient care; V.P.1 Manage appointment schedule, using established priorities; V.P.6 Use office hardware and software to maintain office systems

Name _____   Date _____   Score _____

COMPETENCY ASSESSMENT

Procedure 13-9   Scheduling Inpatient and Outpatient Admissions and Procedures

Task: To assist patients in scheduling inpatient and outpatient admissions and procedures ordered by the provider.

Condition: Calendar, black ink pen, telephone, referral slip, patient's schedule/calendar, provider's requests/orders regarding procedure/admittance, Scenario information

Standards: Perform the Task within 20 minutes with a minimum score of _____ points.

Work Documentation: Documentation of the referral in the patient's chart, with referral slip included

No.	Step	Points	Check #1	Check #2	Check #3
1	Ensure patient understands the inpatient admission or outpatient procedure ordered. If required, seek permission from the patient's insurance company for the procedure or admissions.				
2	Place telephone call to the facility. Identify self, provider, clinic name, and the reason for calling. Identify patient diagnosis and request next available appointment; identify urgency if appropriate.				
3	Confer with the patient regarding appointment time suggested and provide receiver with an immediate affirmative response. Provide receiver with patient information and request special instructions or advanced data.				
4	During call and interaction with patient, demonstrate professional behavior, including: • Demonstrate empathy in communicating with patients, family, and staff • Apply active listening skills • Demonstrate recognition of the patient's level of understanding in communications • Analyze communications in providing appropriate responses/feedback				
5	Complete the referral slip for the patient; send or fax a copy to referred facility.				
6	Appropriately document the referral in the patient's chart; include a copy of the referral slip.				
Student's Total Points					
Points Possible					
Final Score (Student's Total Points/ Possible Points)					

Name _____   Date _____   Score _____

WORK DOCUMENTATION

*Attach referral slips.

_____

Instructor's/Evaluator's Comments and Suggestions:

_____

_____

_____

_____

_____

CHECK #1	
Evaluator's Signature:	Date:

CHECK #2	
Evaluator's Signature:	Date:

CHECK #3	
Evaluator's Signature:	Date:

ABHES Competency: VI.A.1.a.2.e Use proper telephone techniques; VI.A.1.a.2.h Receive, organize, prioritize, and transmit information expediently; VI.A.1.a.3.g schedule inpatient and outpatient admissions

CAAHEP Curriculum: IV.P.2 Report relevant information to others succinctly and accurately; IV.P.7 Demonstrate telephone techniques; V.P.2 Schedule patient admissions and/or procedures

Name _____ **Date** _____ **Score** _____

COMPETENCY ASSESSMENT

Procedure 14-1 Establishing a Paper Medical Chart for a New Patient

Task: To demonstrate an understanding of the principles for establishing a paper medical chart.

Condition: Supplies listed in Procedure 14-6

Standards: Perform the Task within 15 minutes with a minimum score of _____ points.

Work Documentation: Completed paper medical chart

No.	Step	Points	Check #1	Check #2	Check #3
1	Assemble all supplies at a desk or table and prepare them correctly.				
2	Index and code the patient's name according to the filing system to be used. Affix appropriately labeled tabs to the folder cut.				
3	Transfer demographic data in black ink pen or affix office demographic divider sheet.				
4	Affix HIPAA required information, read and signed by patient.				
5	Place prepared chart in proper location.				
6	During procedure, demonstrate time management principles to maintain effective office function.				
	Student's Total Points				
	Points Possible				
	Final Score (Student's Total Points/ Possible Points)				

Name _____ **Date** _____ **Score** _____

WORK DOCUMENTATION

*Attach completed new Patient Chart.

Instructor's/Evaluator's Comments and Suggestions:

_____

_____

_____

_____

_____

CHECK #1

Evaluator's Signature: _____   Date:

CHECK #2

Evaluator's Signature: _____   Date:

CHECK #3

Evaluator's Signature: _____   Date:

ABHES Competency: VI.A.1.a.3.a Perform basic secretarial skills; VI.A.1.a.3.b Prepare and maintain medical records

CAAHEP Curriculum: V.P.3 Organize a patient's medical record

Name _____ **Date** _____ **Score** _____

COMPETENCY ASSESSMENT

Procedure 14-2 Establishing an Electronic Medical Record for a New Patient Using Medical Office Simulation Software (MOSS)

Task: To demonstrate an understanding of the principles for establishing a paper medical chart.

Condition: Supplies listed in Procedure 14-7

Standards: Perform the Task within 15 minutes with a minimum score of _____ points.

Work Documentation: Screen shots of completed tabs in the Patient Registration screen

No.	Step	Points	Check #1	Check #2	Check #3
1	Open MOSS and select the Patient Registration module. Select Add on the Patient Registration dialog box.				
2	Complete the Patient Information tab with correct information (take a screen shot). Click Save.				
3	Complete the Primary Insurance tab with correct information (take a screen shot). Click Save.				
4	Complete the HIPAA tab with correct information (take a screen shot). Click Save.				
5	During procedure, demonstrate time management principles to maintain effective office function.				
Student's Total Points					
Points Possible					
Final Score (Student's Total Points/ Possible Points)					

Name _____   **Date** _____   **Score** _____

WORK DOCUMENTATION

*Attach screen shots of completed tabs in Registration section: Patient Information, Insurance Information, HIPAA.

Instructor's/Evaluator's Comments and Suggestions:

_____

_____

_____

_____

_____

CHECK #1	
Evaluator's Signature:	Date:

CHECK #2	
Evaluator's Signature:	Date:

CHECK #3	
Evaluator's Signature:	Date:

ABHES Competency: VI.A.1.a.3.a Perform basic secretarial skills; VI.A.1.a.3.b Prepare and maintain medical records

CAAHEP Curriculum: V.P.3 Organize a patient's medical record; V.P.5 Execute data management using electronic healthcare records such as the EMR

Name _____   **Date** _____   **Score** _____

COMPETENCY ASSESSMENT

Procedure 14-3   Correcting a Paper Medical Record

Task: To demonstrate the appropriate method to correct an error in a medical chart.

Condition: Scenario information, red ink pen

Standards: Perform this objective within 3 minutes with a minimum score of _____ points.

Work
Documentation: Corrected entry in paper medical record

No.	Step	Points	Check #1	Check #2	Check #3
1	Review information on correction of medical records.				
2	Draw single red line through error.				
3	Write in the correct information.				
4	Follow standard clinic protocol in making the correction: *(options: make "error" or "correction" notation above error or corrected information):* • Demonstrate awareness of the consequences of not working within the legal scope of practice • Recognize the importance of local, state, and federal legislation and regulations in the practice setting				
5	Initial and date the correction.				
Student's Total Points					
Points Possible					
Final Score (Student's Total Points/ Possible Points)					

Name _____   **Date** _____   **Score** _____

WORK DOCUMENTATION

*Attach corrected patient chart entry.

Instructor's/Evaluator's Comments and Suggestions:

_____

_____

_____

_____

_____

CHECK #1
Evaluator's Signature: _____   Date:

CHECK #2
Evaluator's Signature: _____   Date:

CHECK #3
Evaluator's Signature: _____   Date:

ABHES Competency: VI.A.1.a.3.b Prepare and maintain medical records

CAAHEP Curriculum: IX.P.7 Document accurately in the patient record

Name _____ **Date** _____ **Score** _____

COMPETENCY ASSESSMENT

Procedure 14-4 Correcting an Electronic Medical Record

Task: To demonstrate the appropriate method of correction errors in electronic medical records.

Condition: Computer with screen open to document containing error, document containing correction

Standards: Perform the Task within 3 minutes with a minimum score of _____ points.

No.	Step	Points	Check #1	Check #2	Check #3
1	Set the software to track the area to be corrected.				
2	Line out the error using the dash key.				
3	Key in the correction to be made beside the error.				
4	Follow standard clinic protocol in making the correction: *(options: make "error" or "correction" notation above error or corrected information):* • Demonstrate awareness of the consequences of not working within the legal scope of practice • Recognize the importance of local, state, and federal legislation and regulations in the practice setting				
5	Initial and date the correction.				
Student's Total Points					
Points Possible					
Final Score (Student's Total Points/ Possible Points)					

Name _____ **Date** _____ **Score** _____

Instructor's/Evaluator's Comments and Suggestions:

_____

_____

_____

_____

_____

CHECK #1

Evaluator's Signature: _____ Date:

CHECK #2

Evaluator's Signature: _____ Date:

CHECK #3

Evaluator's Signature: _____ Date:

ABHES Competency: VI.A.1.a.3.b Prepare and maintain medical records

CAAHEP Curriculum: IX.P.7 Document accurately in the patient record

Name _____ **Date** _____ **Score** _____

COMPETENCY ASSESSMENT

Procedure 14-5   Steps for Manual Filing with an Alphabetic System

Task: To demonstrate an understanding of the principles of the alphabetic filing system.

Condition: Documents to be filed, dividers with guides, miscellaneous number file section, alphabetic card file and cards, accession journal if needed

Standards: Perform the Task within 15 minutes with a minimum score of _____ points.

No.	Step	Points	Check #1	Check #2	Check #3
1	Inspect and index.				
2	Sort of the charts alphabetically.				
3	Create cross-reference files according to clinic policy.				
4	File the charts appropriately.				
5	Check chart placement to ensure chart is in correct location.				
6	During procedure, demonstrate time management principles to maintain effective office function.				
	Student's Total Points				
	Points Possible				
	Final Score (Student's Total Points/ Possible Points)				

Name _____ **Date** _____ **Score** _____

Instructor's/Evaluator's Comments and Suggestions:

_____

_____

_____

_____

_____

CHECK #1

Evaluator's Signature: _____ Date:

CHECK #2

Evaluator's Signature: _____ Date:

CHECK #3

Evaluator's Signature: _____ Date:

ABHES Competency: VI.A.1.a.3.a Perform basic secretarial skills; VI.A.1.a.3.h File medical records

CAAHEP Curriculum: V.P.4 File medical records; V.P.8 Maintain organization by filing

Name _____ **Date** _____ **Score** _____

COMPETENCY ASSESSMENT

Procedure 14-6   Steps for Manual Filing with a Numeric System

Task: To demonstrate an understanding of the principles of the numeric filing system.

Condition: Documents to be filed, dividers with guides, miscellaneous number file section, alphabetic card file and cards, accession journal if needed

Standards: Perform the Task within 15 minutes with a minimum score of _____ points.

No.	Step	Points	Check #1	Check #2	Check #3
1	Inspect and index.				
2	Code for filing units.				
3	Write the number in the upper-right corner. If no number is assigned, check the miscellaneous file. If item is ready to be assigned, make a card and note number, cross out *M*, and make a chart file.				
4	If there is no card, make up an alphabetic card. Cross-reference if necessary and file the card properly.				
5	File in ascending order.				
6	During procedure, demonstrate time management principles to maintain effective office function.				
Student's Total Points					
Points Possible					
Final Score (Student's Total Points/ Possible Points)					

Name _____   **Date** _____   **Score** _____

Instructor's/Evaluator's Comments and Suggestions:

_____

_____

_____

_____

_____

CHECK #1

Evaluator's Signature: _____   Date:

CHECK #2

Evaluator's Signature: _____   Date:

CHECK #3

Evaluator's Signature: _____   Date:

ABHES Competency: VI.A.1.a.3.a Perform basic secretarial skills; VI.A.1.a.3.h File medical records

CAAHEP Curriculum: V.P.4 File medical records; V.P.8 Maintain organization by filing

Name _____ **Date** _____ **Score** _____

COMPETENCY ASSESSMENT

Procedure 14-7   Steps for Manual Filing with a Subject Filing System

Task: To demonstrate an understanding of the principles of the subject filing system.

Condition: Documents to be filed by subject, subject index list or index card filing listing subjects, alphabetic card file and cards

Standards: Perform the Task within 15 minutes with a minimum score of _____ points.

No.	Step	Points	Check #1	Check #2	Check #3
1	Review the item to find the subject.				
2	Match the subject of the item with an appropriate category. If necessary, decide on proper cross-reference.				
3	Underline any subject title on the material. Write subject title in upper right corner and underline.				
4	Use wavy underline for cross-referencing; use an *X* as with alphabetic and numeric filing.				
5	Underline the first indexing unit.				
6	During procedure, demonstrate time management principles to maintain effective office function.				
Student's Total Points					
Points Possible					
Final Score (Student's Total Points/ Possible Points)					

Name _____   Date _____   Score _____

Instructor's/Evaluator's Comments and Suggestions:

_____

_____

_____

_____

_____

CHECK #1

Evaluator's Signature: Date:

CHECK #2

Evaluator's Signature: Date:

CHECK #3

Evaluator's Signature: Date:

ABHES Competency: VI.A.1.a.3.a Perform basic secretarial skills; VI.A.1.a.3.h File medical records

CAAHEP Curriculum: V.P.4 File medical records; V.P.8 Maintain organization by filing

Name _____ Date _____ Score _____

COMPETENCY ASSESSMENT

Procedure 15-1   Preparing and Composing Business Correspondence Using All Components (Computerized Approach)

Task: To prepare and compose a final copy letter using appropriate language and letter style to convey a clear and accurate message to the recipient.

Condition: Supplies listed in Procedure 15-1

Standards: Perform the Task within 20 minutes with a minimum score of _____ points.

Work Documentation: Completed, printed letter

No.	Step	Points	Check #1	Check #2	Check #3
1	Open word processing program. Set margins and other layout parameters, choose and set fonts. Save the document.				
2	Compose a rough outline/draft of the letter. Correct any errors. Save the document.				
3	Using the appropriate letter style, type the date, recipient's name and address, salutation, subject of the letter, body of the letter, complimentary closing, signature line, reference, and enclosure notations.				
4	Select language that demonstrates recognition of the patient's level of understanding in communications.				
5	Proofread the document and make corrections as appropriate. Save the document.				
6	Print two copies of the document. Prepare the letter, with envelope, for the provider's review and signature. File the other copy appropriately.				
Student's Total Points					
Points Possible					
Final Score (Student's Total Points/ Possible Points)					

Name _____ **Date** _____ **Score** _____

WORK DOCUMENTATION

*Attach printed letter.

_____

Instructor's/Evaluator's Comments and Suggestions:

_____
_____
_____
_____
_____

CHECK #1

Evaluator's Signature: _____   Date:

CHECK #2

Evaluator's Signature: _____   Date:

CHECK #3

Evaluator's Signature: _____   Date:

ABHES Competency: VI.A.1.a.2.j Use correct grammar, spelling, and formatting techniques in written works; VI.A.1.a.2.o Fundamental writing skills

CAAHEP Curriculum: V.P.10 Compose professional/business letters

Name _____ **Date** _____ **Score** _____

COMPETENCY ASSESSMENT

Procedure 15-2   Addressing Envelopes According to United States Postal Regulations

Task: To address envelopes according to U.S. Postal Service regulations to ensure timely delivery.

Condition: Supplies listed in Procedure 15-2

Standards: Perform the Task within 5 minutes with a minimum score of _____ points.

Work Documentation: Completed envelope

No.	Step	Points	Check #1	Check #2	Check #3
1	Select the envelope format from the software program, or use labels.				
2	Place the address within the proper area as directed by the U.S. postal regulations.				
3	Key the address correctly. If not using preprinted envelopes, key the return address correctly.				
4	Proofread the envelope; make corrections as necessary.				
Student's Total Points					
Points Possible					
Final Score (Student's Total Points/ Possible Points)					

Name _____   **Date** _____   **Score** _____

WORK DOCUMENTATION
*Attach completed envelope.

_____

Instructor's/Evaluator's Comments and Suggestions:

_____

_____

_____

_____

_____

CHECK #1

Evaluator's Signature: _____   Date:

CHECK #2

Evaluator's Signature: _____   Date:

CHECK #3

Evaluator's Signature: _____   Date:

ABHES Competency: VI.A.1.a.3.a Perform basic secretarial skills

Name _____   **Date** _____   **Score** _____

COMPETENCY ASSESSMENT

Procedure 15-3   Folding Letters for Standard Envelopes

Task: To fold and insert letters into envelopes so that the letters fit properly in the envelopes.

Condition: Supplies listed in Procedure 15-3

Standards: Perform the Task within 2 minutes with a minimum score of _____ points.

No.	Step	Points	Check #1	Check #2	Check #3
1	Fold letter to fit into a number 6¾ envelope.				
2	Fold letter to fit into a number 10 envelope.				
3	Fold letter to fit into a window envelope.				
Student's Total Points					
Points Possible					
Final Score (Student's Total Points/ Possible Points)					

Name _____   **Date** _____   **Score** _____

Instructor's/Evaluator's Comments and Suggestions:

_____

_____

_____

_____

_____

CHECK #1

Evaluator's Signature: Date:

CHECK #2

Evaluator's Signature: Date:

CHECK #3

Evaluator's Signature: Date:

ABHES Competency: VI.A.1.a.3.a Perform basic secretarial skills

Name _____   **Date** _____   **Score** _____

COMPETENCY ASSESSMENT

Procedure 15-4   Creating a Mass Mailing Using Mail Merge

Task: To create a mass mailing using the computer's Mail Merge Helper feature contained within Microsoft® Word.

Condition: Supplies listed in Procedure 15-4

Standards: Perform the Task within 15 minutes with a minimum score of _____ points.

No.	Step	Points	Check #1	Check #2	Check #3
1	Compose and type the document.				
2	Develop a data source.				
3	Insert merge fields into the main document.				
4	Send the merged document to the printer.				
Student's Total Points					
Points Possible					
Final Score (Student's Total Points/ Possible Points)					

Name _____   **Date** _____   **Score** _____

Instructor's/Evaluator's Comments and Suggestions:

_____

_____

_____

_____

_____

CHECK #1

Evaluator's Signature: _____   Date:

CHECK #2

Evaluator's Signature: _____   Date:

CHECK #3

Evaluator's Signature: _____   Date:

ABHES Competency: VI.A.1.a.3.a Perform basic secretarial skills; VI.A.1.a.3.d Apply computer concepts for office procedures

Name _____   **Date** _____   **Score** _____

COMPETENCY ASSESSMENT

Procedure 15-5   Preparing Outgoing Mail According to United States Postal Regulations

Task: To prepare outgoing mail for expeditious delivery.

Condition: Supplies listed in Procedure 15-5

Standards: Perform the Task within 15 minutes with a minimum score of _____ points.

No.	Step	Points	Check #1	Check #2	Check #3
1	Sort the mail according to postal class.				
2	Weigh the item to be mailed.				
3	Affix the appropriate postage.				
4	Place item(s) in outgoing mail, or deliver to post office.				
Student's Total Points					
Points Possible					
Final Score (Student's Total Points/ Possible Points)					

Name _____ **Date** _____ **Score** _____

Instructor's/Evaluator's Comments and Suggestions:

_____

_____

_____

_____

_____

CHECK #1

Evaluator's Signature: _____ Date: _____

CHECK #2

Evaluator's Signature: _____ Date: _____

CHECK #3

Evaluator's Signature: _____ Date: _____

ABHES Competency: VI.A.1.a.3.a Perform basic secretarial skills

Name _____   **Date** _____   **Score** _____

COMPETENCY ASSESSMENT

Procedure 17-1 Applying Managed Care Policies and Procedures

Task: To apply managed care policies and procedures that the provider and/or medical facility has partnership agreements with.

Condition: Managed care contracts, managed care policies and procedures manuals, patient record, authorized forms from managed care organizations, clerical supplies

Standards: Perform the Task within 15 minutes with a minimum score of _____ points.

Work
Documentation: Entry in patient's medical record

No.	Step	Points	Check #1	Check #2	Check #3
1	Called insurance company and obtained the correct information, including: • Verified patient has insurance in effect and was eligible for benefits • Confirmed exclusions and noncovered services • Determined deductibles, copayments or other payments the patient is responsible for • Inquired about preauthorizations • Used appropriate telephone techniques during call • Documented the name, title, and extension of person contacted				
2	Collected information from patient, and correctly documented the information collected.				
3	During procedure, demonstrated professional behavior in manner, organization, and attire.				
	Student's Total Points				
	Points Possible				
	Final Score (Student's Total Points/ Possible Points)				

Name _____   Date _____   Score _____

WORK DOCUMENTATION

Instructor's/Evaluator's Comments and Suggestions:

_____

_____

_____

_____

_____

CHECK #1

Evaluator's Signature: _____   Date:

CHECK #2

Evaluator's Signature: _____   Date:

CHECK #3

Evaluator's Signature: _____   Date:

ABHES Competency: VI.A.1.a.3.t Apply managed care policies and procedures; VI.A.1.a.8.c Analyze and use current third-party guidelines for reimbursement

CAAHEP Curriculum: VII.P.1 Apply both managed care policies and procedures; VII.P.2 Apply third party guidelines; VII.P.6 Verify eligibility for managed care services

Name _____   **Date** _____   **Score** _____

COMPETENCY ASSESSMENT

Procedure 17-2   Screening for Insurance

Task: To verify insurance coverage and obtain vital information required for processing and billing insurance claim forms.

Condition: Patient registration forms, clipboard and black ink pen, patient's chart

Standards: Perform the Task within 15 minutes with a minimum score of _____ points.

No.	Step	Points	Check #1	Check #2	Check #3
1	Ask patients to bring their insurance cards and arrive 15–20 minutes before appointment time.				
2	Review completed patient registration form for legibility and completeness. Verify address and insurance coverage; check insurance card; determine that primary care provider is performing the procedure and that the procedure is covered; determine if referral is needed.				
3	Make front and back photocopies of patient's insurance card and attach to patient's chart. Verify proof of eligibility for Medicaid patients.				
4	During interaction with patient, demonstrate professional behavior, including: • Demonstrate sensitivity in communicating with patient • Communicate in language the patient can understand regarding managed care and insurance plans				
	Student's Total Points				
	Points Possible				
	Final Score (Student's Total Points/ Possible Points)				

Name _____   **Date** _____   **Score** _____

Instructor's/Evaluator's Comments and Suggestions:

_____

_____

_____

_____

_____

CHECK #1

Evaluator's Signature: _____   Date:

CHECK #2

Evaluator's Signature: _____   Date:

CHECK #3

Evaluator's Signature: _____   Date:

ABHES Competency: VI.A.1.a.3.t Apply managed care policies and procedures; VI.A.1.a.8.c Analyze and use current third-party guidelines for reimbursement

CAAHEP Curriculum: VII.P.1 Apply both managed care policies and procedures; VII.P.2 Apply third party guidelines; VII.P.6 Verify eligibility for managed care services

Name _____   **Date** _____   **Score** _____

COMPETENCY ASSESSMENT

Procedure 17-3   Obtaining Referrals and Authorizations

Task: To ascertain coverage by the insurance carrier for specific medical services, hospital admissions, inpatient or outpatient surgeries, elective procedures, or when the primary care provider elects to refer the patient to another provider.

Condition: Patient's medical chart and copy of the patient's insurance card, name of the carrier contact person and telephone number, completed referral form, telephone/fax machine, pen/pencil

Standards: Perform the Task within 15 minutes with a minimum score of _____ points.

Work
Documentation: Completed copy of the referral form

No.	Step	Points	Check #1	Check #2	Check #3
1	Collect all necessary documents and equipment. Determine the service or procedure requiring preauthorization.				
2	Complete and proofread the referral form. Use language that demonstrates assertive communication with managed care and/or insurance providers.				
3	Fax the completed form to the insurance carrier. Maintain a completed copy of the referral form in the patient's chart.				
4	Maintain a completed copy of the authorization number/code in the patient's chart.				
Student's Total Points					
Points Possible					
Final Score (Student's Total Points/ Possible Points)					

Name _____ **Date** _____ **Score** _____

WORK DOCUMENTATION
*Attach completed referral form.

_____

Instructor's/Evaluator's Comments and Suggestions:

_____

_____

_____

_____

_____

CHECK #1	
Evaluator's Signature:	Date:

CHECK #2	
Evaluator's Signature:	Date:

CHECK #3	
Evaluator's Signature:	Date:

ABHES Competency: VI.A.1.a.3.t Apply managed care policies and procedures; VI.A.1.a.3.u Obtain managed care referrals and pre-certification; VI.A.1.a.8.c Analyze and use current third-party guidelines for reimbursement

CAAHEP Curriculum: VII.P.4 Obtain precertification, including documentation; VII.P.5 Obtain preauthorization, including documentation

Name _____   **Date** _____   **Score** _____

COMPETENCY ASSESSMENT

Procedure 17-4   Computing the Medicare Fee Schedule

Task: To compute the Medicare allowable (MA) payment for services.

Condition: CPT book, computer, calculator

Standards: Perform the Task within 15 minutes with a minimum score of _____ points.

Work Documentation: Calculation and correct answer in the Work Documentation area

No.	Step	Points	Check #1	Check #2	Check #3
1	Obtained the correct CPT code for the procedure or service performed.				
2	Used the Medicare Fee Schedule and correctly determined the Medicare allowable fee: • Determined each value of the allowable formula • Used the formula correctly to calculate the fee • Correctly rounded, if appropriate				
	Student's Total Points				
	Points Possible				
	Final Score (Student's Total Points/ Possible Points)				

Name _____ **Date** _____ **Score** _____

WORK DOCUMENTATION

_____

Instructor's/Evaluator's Comments and Suggestions:

_____

_____

_____

_____

_____

CHECK #1

Evaluator's Signature: _____   Date:

CHECK #2

Evaluator's Signature: _____   Date:

CHECK #3

Evaluator's Signature: _____   Date:

ABHES Competency: VI.A.1.a.3.t Apply managed care policies and procedures

CAAHEP Curriculum: VII.P.1 Apply both managed care policies and procedures

Name _____ **Date** _____ **Score** _____

COMPETENCY ASSESSMENT

Procedure 18-1   Current Procedural Terminology Coding

Task: To convert commonly accepted descriptions of medical procedures (services) and for visits of all kinds—office, hospital, nursing facility, home services—into a five-digit numeric code with two-digit numeric modifiers when required.

Condition: CPT code book for the current year; copy of the encounter form and access to the patient's chart, pencil and paper; Scenario information

Standards: Perform the Task within 15 minutes with a minimum score of _____ points.

Work Documentation: Correct code selection in Work Documentation section

No.	Step	Points	Check #1	Check #2	Check #3
1	Using the CPT code book and the Scenario information, find the correct E&M service code.				
2	In the Index, find the correct code for the procedure.				
3	Now locate the code you have found in Step 2 in the Pathology and Laboratory section; ensure the description provided matches what the provider has documented in the patient's chart.				
Student's Total Points					
Points Possible					
Final Score (Student's Total Points/ Possible Points)					

Name _____ **Date** _____ **Score** _____

WORK DOCUMENTATION

Enter correct code:

_____

Instructor's/Evaluator's Comments and Suggestions:

_____

_____

_____

_____

_____

CHECK #1	
Evaluator's Signature:	Date:

CHECK #2	
Evaluator's Signature:	Date:

CHECK #3	
Evaluator's Signature:	Date:

ABHES Competency: VI.A.1.a.8.b Implement current procedural terminology and ICD-9 coding

CAAHEP Curriculum: VIII.P.1 Perform procedural coding

Name _____ **Date** _____ **Score** _____

COMPETENCY ASSESSMENT

Procedure 18-2   International Classification of Diseases, 9th Revision, Clinical Modification Coding

Task: The ICD-9-CM code books provide a diagnostic coding system for the compilation and reporting of morbidity and mortality statistics for reimbursement purposes.

Condition: Volumes 1 and 2 of the ICD-9-CM code books for the current year, copy of the encounter form and access to the patient's chart, pencil and paper

Standards: Perform the Task within 15 minutes with a minimum score of _____ points.

*Work
Documentation:* Correct code selection in Work Documentation section

No.	Step	Points	Check #1	Check #2	Check #3
1	Using Volume II of the ICD-9-CM code books, look up the main reason or condition that brought the patient to the facility, or the specific diagnosis confirmed by test results.				
2	Using Volume I, look up the code you found in Step 1. Read all listings and determine the appropriate code having the greatest level of specificity.				
Student's Total Points					
Points Possible					
Final Score (Student's Total Points/ Possible Points)					

Name _____ **Date** _____ **Score** _____

WORK DOCUMENTATION

Enter correct code:

_____

Instructor's/Evaluator's Comments and Suggestions:

_____

_____

_____

_____

_____

CHECK #1

Evaluator's Signature: _____ Date: _____

CHECK #2

Evaluator's Signature: _____ Date: _____

CHECK #3

Evaluator's Signature: _____ Date: _____

ABHES Competency: VI.A.1.a.3.v Perform diagnostic coding; VI.A.1.a.8.b Implement current procedural terminology and ICD-9 coding

CAAHEP Curriculum: VIII.P.2 Perform diagnostic coding

Name _____   **Date** _____   **Score** _____

COMPETENCY ASSESSMENT

Procedure 18-3   Applying Third-Party Guidelines

Task: To obtain written authorization to release necessary medical information to third-party payers.

Condition: Patient chart, CMS-1500 claim form

Standards: Perform the Task within 5 minutes with a minimum score of _____ points.

Work Documentation: Completed CMS-1500 claim form in Work Documentation section

No.	Step	Points	Check #1	Check #2	Check #3
1	When patient signs in, check her/his chart to ascertain if an "Authorization to Release Medical Information" has been signed and is currently valid.				
2	During interaction with patient, demonstrate professional behavior, including: • Communicating in language the patient can understand regarding managed care and insurance plans				
3	If there is no record of signature on file, have the patient sign Block 12 of the CMS-1500 form.				
Student's Total Points					
Points Possible					
Final Score (Student's Total Points/ Possible Points)					

Name _____   **Date** _____   **Score** _____

WORK DOCUMENTATION

*Attach Block 12 of CMS-1500 form.

_____

Instructor's/Evaluator's Comments and Suggestions:

_____
_____
_____
_____
_____

CHECK #1	
Evaluator's Signature:	Date:

CHECK #2	
Evaluator's Signature:	Date:

CHECK #3	
Evaluator's Signature:	Date:

ABHES Competency: VI.A.1.a.3.v Perform diagnostic coding; VI.A.1.a.8.b Implement current procedural terminology and ICD-9 coding

CAAHEP Curriculum: VII.P.2 Apply third party guidelines

Name _____   **Date** _____   **Score** _____

COMPETENCY ASSESSMENT

Procedure 18-4   Completing a Medicare CMS-1500 (08-05) Claim Form

Task: To complete the CMS-1500 insurance claim form for reimbursement.

Condition: Patient information, patient account or ledger card, copy of patient's insurance card, insurance claim form, computer and printer

Standards: Perform the Task within 30 minutes with a minimum score of _____ points.

Work
Documentation: Completed CMS-1500 form

No.	Step	Points	Check #1	Check #2	Check #3
1	Correctly complete the Carrier section, in the upper portion of the form.				
2	Correctly complete the Patient and Insured section of the form, Blocks 1–13.				
3	Correctly complete the Physician or Supplier section of the form, Blocks 14–33.				
4	Proofread the form to ensure information is correct.				
Student's Total Points					
Points Possible					
Final Score (Student's Total Points/ Possible Points)					

Name _____   **Date** _____   **Score** _____

WORK DOCUMENTATION
*Attach completed CMS-1500 form.

_____

Instructor's/Evaluator's Comments and Suggestions:

_____

_____

_____

_____

_____

CHECK #1

Evaluator's Signature: _____   Date:

CHECK #2

Evaluator's Signature: _____   Date:

CHECK #3

Evaluator's Signature: _____   Date:

ABHES Competency: VI.A.1.a.3.v Perform diagnostic coding; VI.A.1.a.3.w Complete insurance claim forms; VI.A.1.a.8.b Implement current procedural terminology and ICD-9 coding

CAAHEP Curriculum: VIII.P.2 Perform diagnostic coding

Name _____ **Date** _____ **Score** _____

COMPETENCY ASSESSMENT

Procedure 19-1   Recording/Posting Patient Charges, Payments, and Adjustments in a Manual System

Task: To record information including services rendered, fees charged, any adjustments made, and balances pertaining to a patient's visit to the provider's and the patient's account.

Condition: Calculator, patient's account or ledger, day sheet

Standards: Perform the Task within 15 minutes with a minimum score of _____ points.

Work Documentation: Completed patient ledger and day sheet

No.	Step	Points	Check #1	Check #2	Check #3
1	Prior to the patient's appointment, check the patient's account to ensure it is current.				
2	When the patient arrives, confirm that all demographic and insurance information is current. Prepare the encounter form with this information.				
3	After the patient's visit, correctly enter the charges on the patient's encounter form and calculate totals.				
4	Correctly record all patient charges, payments, and adjustments to the manual pegboard system.				
5	Enter patient's payment on the day sheet. Place a restrictive endorsement on any checks received and place payment in an appointed secure place awaiting deposit.				
6	During interaction with patient, demonstrate professional behavior, manner, organization, and sensitivity.				
Student's Total Points					
Points Possible					
Final Score (Student's Total Points/ Possible Points)					

Name _____   **Date** _____   **Score** _____

WORK DOCUMENTATION
*Attach completed patient ledger and day sheet.

Instructor's/Evaluator's Comments and Suggestions:

_____

_____

_____

_____

_____

CHECK #1

Evaluator's Signature: _____   Date:

CHECK #2

Evaluator's Signature: _____   Date:

CHECK #3

Evaluator's Signature: _____   Date:

ABHES Competency: VI.A.1.a.3.k Post entries on a day sheet; VI.A.1.a.3.l Perform billing and collection procedures; VI.A.1.a.3.o Post adjustments; VI.A.1.a.8.a Use manual and computerized bookkeeping systems

CAAHEP Curriculum: VI.P.2.a Post entries on a daysheet; VI.P.2.b Perform billing procedures; VI.P.2.d Post adjustments

Name _____ **Date** _____ **Score** _____

COMPETENCY ASSESSMENT

Procedure 19-2   Balancing Day Sheets in a Manual System

Task: To verify that all entries to the day sheet are correct and that the totals balance.

Condition: Day sheet, calculator

Standards: Perform the Task within 15 minutes with a minimum score of _____ points.

*Work
Documentation:*   Completed day sheet

No.	Step	Points	Check #1	Check #2	Check #3
1	Total columns A, B1, B2, C, and D and enter in appropriate fields.				
2	Correctly complete Proof of Posting box.				
3	Correctly complete Accounts Receivable Control box.				
4	Correctly complete Accounts Receivable Proof box.				
5	Correctly calculate the Total Deposit and enter in the appropriate field.				
6	Correctly prepare the next Day Sheet by entering the Previous Day and Month to Date fields.				
Student's Total Points					
Points Possible					
Final Score (Student's Total Points/ Possible Points)					

Name _____ **Date** _____ **Score** _____

WORK DOCUMENTATION

*Attach completed day sheet.

Instructor's/Evaluator's Comments and Suggestions:

_____

_____

_____

_____

_____

CHECK #1

Evaluator's Signature: _____   Date:

CHECK #2

Evaluator's Signature: _____   Date:

CHECK #3

Evaluator's Signature: _____   Date:

ABHES Competency: VI.A.1.a.3.k Post entries on a day sheet; VI.A.1.a.8.a Use manual and computerized bookkeeping systems

CAAHEP Curriculum: VI.P.2.a Post entries on a daysheet

Name _____ **Date** _____ **Score** _____

COMPETENCY ASSESSMENT

Procedure 19-3   Posting Patient Charges Using Medical Office Simulation Software (MOSS)

Task: To electronically post charges to a patient's account.

Condition: Computer, MOSS, Scenario information

Standards: Perform the Task within 15 minutes with a minimum score of _____ points.

Work Documentation: Screen shot of completed Procedure Posting screens

No.	Step	Points	Check #1	Check #2	Check #3
1	Open MOSS and select Procedure Posting from the Main Menu.				
2	Find Jordan Connell in the patient menu and correctly Post all of the charges from his visit (take a screen shot of the completed Procedure Posting screen after all the procedures have been entered).				
3	Find Edward Gormann in the patient menu and correctly Post all of the charges from his visit (take a screen shot of the completed Procedure Posting screen after all the procedures have been entered).				
4	Find Elane Ybarra in the patient menu and correctly Post all of the charges from her visit (take a screen shot of the completed Procedure Posting screen after all the procedures have been entered).				
	Student's Total Points				
	Points Possible				
	Final Score (Student's Total Points/ Possible Points)				

Name _____   Date _____   Score _____

WORK DOCUMENTATION

*Attach screen shots of completed Procedure Posting screens.

Instructor's/Evaluator's Comments and Suggestions:

_____

_____

_____

_____

_____

CHECK #1

Evaluator's Signature: _____   Date: _____

CHECK #2

Evaluator's Signature: _____   Date: _____

CHECK #3

Evaluator's Signature: _____   Date: _____

ABHES Competency: VI.A.1.a.3.d Apply computer concepts for office procedures; VI.A.1.a.3.l Perform billing and collection procedures; VI.A.1.a.8.a Use manual and computerized bookkeeping systems

CAAHEP Curriculum: VI.P.2.b Perform billing procedures; VI.P.3 Utilize computerized office billing systems

Name _____   **Date** _____   **Score** _____

COMPETENCY ASSESSMENT

Procedure 19-4   Insurance Billing Using Medical Office Simulation Software (MOSS)

Task: To complete the CMS-1500 insurance claim form for reimbursement using a computerized system.

Condition: MOSS, computer, printer, Scenario information

Standards: Perform the Task within 15 minutes with a minimum score of _____ points.

Work Documentation: Printed pre-billing worksheet; printed transmission report

No.	Step	Points	Check #1	Check #2	Check #3
1	Open MOSS and select the Insurance Billing module from the Main Menu.				
2	Correctly complete the Claims Preparation screen for Jordan Connell.				
3	Click on the Prebilling Worksheet button and verify information is correct; print this report for Jordan Connell and close.				
4	Select Generate Claims and verify CMS-1500 form is correct; select transmit EMC to send the report to the payer. Print the transmission status report for Jordan Connell and close.				
5	Following the same steps, transmit a claim for Edward Gormann. Print prebilling worksheet and transmission report.				
6	Following the same steps, transmit a claim for Elane Ybarra. Print prebilling worksheet and transmission report.				
Student's Total Points					
Points Possible					
Final Score (Student's Total Points/ Possible Points)					

Name _____ **Date** _____ **Score** _____

WORK DOCUMENTATION

*Attach pre-billing worksheets and transmission reports.

_____

Instructor's/Evaluator's Comments and Suggestions:

_____

_____

_____

_____

_____

CHECK #1

Evaluator's Signature: _____ Date:

CHECK #2

Evaluator's Signature: _____ Date:

CHECK #3

Evaluator's Signature: _____ Date:

ABHES Competency: VI.A.1.a.3.d Apply computer concepts for office procedures; VI.A.1.a.3.w Complete insurance claim forms

CAAHEP Curriculum: VI.P.3 Utilize computerized office billing systems; VII.P.3 Complete insurance claim forms

Name _____   **Date** _____   **Score** _____

COMPETENCY ASSESSMENT

Procedure 19-5   Posting Payments and Adjustments Using Medical Office Simulation Software (MOSS)

Task: To post insurance payments and adjustments electronically.

Condition: Computer, MOSS, Scenario information

Standards: Perform the Task within 15 minutes with a minimum score of _____ points.

Work Documentation: Screen shot of completed Payment Posting screens

No.	Step	Points	Check #1	Check #2	Check #3
1	Open MOSS and select Posting Payments from the Main Menu.				
2	Find Edward Gormann in the patient menu and correctly Post all insurance payments and adjustments (take a screen shot of the completed Payment Posting screen after all the payments and adjustments have been entered).				
3	Find Jordan Connell in the patient menu and correctly Post all insurance payments and adjustments (take a screen shot of the completed Payment Posting screen after all the payments and adjustments have been entered).				
4	Find Elane Ybarra in the patient menu and correctly Post all insurance payments and adjustments (take a screen shot of the completed Payment Posting screen after all the payments and adjustments have been entered).				
Student's Total Points					
Points Possible					
Final Score (Student's Total Points/ Possible Points)					

Name _____   **Date** _____   **Score** _____

WORK DOCUMENTATION

*Attach screen shots of completed Payment Posting screens.

_____

Instructor's/Evaluator's Comments and Suggestions:

_____

_____

_____

_____

_____

CHECK #1	
Evaluator's Signature:	Date:

CHECK #2	
Evaluator's Signature:	Date:

CHECK #3	
Evaluator's Signature:	Date:

ABHES Competency: VI.A.1.a.3.d Apply computer concepts for office procedures; VI.A.1.a.3.l Perform billing and collection procedures; VI.A.1.a.3.o Post adjustments; VI.A.1.a.8.a Use manual and computerized bookkeeping systems

CAAHEP Curriculum: VI.P.2.c Perform collection procedures; VI.P.2.d Post adjustments; VI.P.3 Utilize computerized office billing systems

Name _____ Date _____ Score _____

COMPETENCY ASSESSMENT

Procedure 19-6   Processing Credit Balances and Refunds Using Medical Office Simulation Software (MOSS)

Task:　　　　　To process credit balances and refunds electronically.

Condition:　　Computer, MOSS, Scenario information

Standards:　　Perform the Task within 15 minutes with a minimum score of _____ points.

Work Documentation:　Screen shot of completed Payment Posting screens

No.	Step	Points	Check #1	Check #2	Check #3
1	Open MOSS and select Posting Payments from the Main Menu.				
2	Find Josephine Albertson in the patient menu and correctly process her refund and click Post (take a screen shot of the completed Payment Posting screen).				
3	Find Andrew Jefferson in the patient menu and select correctly process his overpayment and click Post (take a screen shot of the completed Payment Posting screen).				
4	Find Alice Maxwell in the patient menu and correctly process her refund and click Post (take a screen shot of the completed Payment Posting screen).				
Student's Total Points					
Points Possible					
Final Score (Student's Total Points/ Possible Points)					

Name _____ **Date** _____ **Score** _____

WORK DOCUMENTATION

*Attach screen shots of completed Payment Posting screens.

_____

Instructor's/Evaluator's Comments and Suggestions:

_____

_____

_____

_____

_____

CHECK #1	
Evaluator's Signature:	Date:

CHECK #2	
Evaluator's Signature:	Date:

CHECK #3	
Evaluator's Signature:	Date:

ABHES Competency: VI.A.1.a.3.d Apply computer concepts for office procedures; VI.A.1.a.3.p Process credit balance; VI.A.1.a.3.p Process refunds; VI.A.1.a.8.a Use manual and computerized bookkeeping systems

CAAHEP Curriculum: VI.P.2.e Process a credit balance; VI.P.2.f Process refunds; VI.P.3 Utilize computerized office billing systems

Name _____   Date _____   Score _____

COMPETENCY ASSESSMENT

Procedure 19-7   Preparing a Deposit

Task: To create a deposit slip for the day's receipts.

Condition: Deposit slip, check endorsement stamp, calculator, cash and checks received for the day, day sheet

Standards: Perform the Task within 15 minutes with a minimum score of _____ points.

Work Documentation: Completed deposit slip

No.	Step	Points	Check #1	Check #2	Check #3
1	Separate cash from checks.				
2	Prepare bills and coins properly, following bank procedure. Correctly count all cash and currency and enter the totals in the appropriate fields on the deposit slip.				
3	Correctly enter each check separately on the back of the deposit slip, and copy the total to the front of the deposit slip in the appropriate field.				
4	Correctly complete the front of the deposit slip. Compare the total the cash and currency to the day sheet total to ensure they are the same.				
5	Enter the deposit information in the checkbook stub and checkbook balance.				
6	Make the deposit at the bank, and get a receipt for the office's records.				
Student's Total Points					
Points Possible					
Final Score (Student's Total Points/ Possible Points)					

Name _____   Date _____   Score _____

WORK DOCUMENTATION

*Attach completed deposit slip.

_____

Instructor's/Evaluator's Comments and Suggestions:

_____

_____

_____

_____

_____

CHECK #1

Evaluator's Signature: _____   Date:

CHECK #2

Evaluator's Signature: _____   Date:

CHECK #3

Evaluator's Signature: _____   Date:

ABHES Competency: VI.A.1.a.3.i Prepare a bank statement and deposit record

CAAHEP Curriculum: VI.P.1 Prepare a bank deposit

Name _____   **Date** _____   **Score** _____

COMPETENCY ASSESSMENT

Procedure 19-8 Recording a Nonsufficient Funds Check in a Manual System

Task: To record a NSF check, performing bookkeeping a function that keeps account in proper balance.

Condition: The practice's account balance, day sheet, patient ledger, NSF check

Standards: Perform the Task within 15 minutes with a minimum score of _____ points.

Work Documentation: Completed day sheet and patient ledger

No.	Step	Points	Check #1	Check #2	Check #3
1	Follow policy for notifying the patient of NSF check. When the NSF has been returned a second time, deduct the check amount from the account balance of the practice.				
2	Correctly add the amount of the NSF back into the patient's ledger, enter the explanation in the description column, and update the total.				
Student's Total Points					
Points Possible					
Final Score (Student's Total Points/ Possible Points)					

Name _____   **Date** _____   **Score** _____

WORK DOCUMENTATION
*Attach completed day sheet and ledger.

_____

Instructor's/Evaluator's Comments and Suggestions:

_____

_____

_____

_____

_____

CHECK #1	
Evaluator's Signature:	Date:

CHECK #2	
Evaluator's Signature:	Date:

CHECK #3	
Evaluator's Signature:	Date:

ABHES Competency: VI.A.1.a.3.r Post NSF funds
CAAHEP Curriculum: VI.P.2.g Post non-sufficient fund (NSF) checks

Name _____   **Date** _____   **Score** _____

COMPETENCY ASSESSMENT

Procedure 19-9   Writing a Check

Task: To write a check to pay for expenses incurred and provide proof of payment.

Condition: Check Writing Exercises 1–5 in Procedure 19-11, checkbook, check register, pen with black ink, calculator

Standards: Perform the Task within 15 minutes with a minimum score of _____ points.

Work Documentation: Completed checks and check registers

No.	Step	Points	Check #1	Check #2	Check #3
1	Gather all invoices (Check Writing Exercises). Correctly complete the check register and check for Check Writing Exercise 1.				
2	Correctly complete the check register and check for Check Writing Exercise 2.				
3	Correctly complete the check register and check for Check Writing Exercise 3.				
4	Correctly complete the check register and check for Check Writing Exercise 4.				
5	Correctly complete the check register and check for Check Writing Exercise 5.				
Student's Total Points					
Points Possible					
Final Score (Student's Total Points/ Possible Points)					

Name _____   **Date** _____   **Score** _____

WORK DOCUMENTATION

*Attach completed checks.

Instructor's/Evaluator's Comments and Suggestions:

_____

_____

_____

_____

_____

CHECK #1

Evaluator's Signature: _____   Date:

CHECK #2

Evaluator's Signature: _____   Date:

CHECK #3

Evaluator's Signature: _____   Date:

ABHES Competency: VI.A.1.a.3.m Prepare a check; VI.A.1.a.6.a Maintain physical plant

Name _____   **Date** _____   **Score** _____

COMPETENCY ASSESSMENT

Procedure 19-10 Reconciling a Bank Statement

Task: To verify that the balance listed in the checkbook agrees with the balance shown by the bank.

Condition: Checkbook, bank statement, calculator

Standards: Perform the Task within 15 minutes with a minimum score of _____ points.

Work Documentation: Completed bank statement worksheet

No.	Step	Points	Check #1	Check #2	Check #3
1	Make sure the balance in the checkbook is correct, and that any service charge from the bank is subtracted from the current balance listed in the checkbook.				
2	In the checkbook, check off each check listed on the statement. Then, check off each deposit listed on the statement.				
3	Determine the totals of checks not cleared and deposits not credited, and enter the totals on the bank statement worksheet.				
4	Correctly complete the remainder of the bank statement worksheet, performing the appropriate calculations.				
5	The total on the bank statement worksheet equals the balance in the checkbook. File the bank statement appropriately.				
Student's Total Points					
Points Possible					
Final Score (Student's Total Points/ Possible Points)					

Name _____ **Date** _____ **Score** _____

WORK DOCUMENTATION
*Attach completed bank statement worksheet.

_____

Instructor's/Evaluator's Comments and Suggestions:

_____

_____

_____

_____

_____

CHECK #1

Evaluator's Signature: _____   Date:

CHECK #2

Evaluator's Signature: _____   Date:

CHECK #3

Evaluator's Signature: _____   Date:

ABHES Competency: VI.A.1.a.3.j Reconcile a bank statement; VI.A.1.a.8.e Maintain records for accounting and banking purposes

Name _____   **Date** _____   **Score** _____

COMPETENCY ASSESSMENT

Procedure 19-11   Establishing and Maintaining a Petty Cash Fund

Task: To establish and maintain a petty cash fund for incidental expenses making certain that receipts match the difference between the beginning and ending balance of the fund.

Condition: Petty Cash Exercises listed in Procedure 19-9, blank check, cash box, calculator

Standards: Perform the Task within 15 minutes with a minimum score of _____ points.

Work Documentation: Two completed checks

No.	Step	Points	Check #1	Check #2	Check #3
1	Correctly prepare a check for $100, written to "Cash."				
2	Receive the cash and place in cash box.				
3	Using the Petty Cash Exercises, correctly prepare vouchers for the amounts needed. Remove the appropriate cash from the cash box.				
4	After the purchases, place receipts for the purchases in the cash box.				
5	Correctly balance the Petty Cash fund by counting the money remaining and totaling the receipts.				
6	Correctly prepare a check for the amount that was used, bringing the total of the Petty Cash fund back to $100.				
Student's Total Points					
Points Possible					
Final Score (Student's Total Points/ Possible Points)					

Name _____ **Date** _____ **Score** _____

WORK DOCUMENTATION

*Attach completed checks.

Instructor's/Evaluator's Comments and Suggestions:

_____

_____

_____

_____

_____

CHECK #1

Evaluator's Signature: _____ Date: _____

CHECK #2

Evaluator's Signature: _____ Date: _____

CHECK #3

Evaluator's Signature: _____ Date: _____

ABHES Competency: VI.A.1.a.3.m Prepare a check; VI.A.1.a.3.n Establish and maintain a petty cash fund

Name _____   **Date** _____   **Score** _____

COMPETENCY ASSESSMENT

Procedure 20-1   Explaining Fees in the First Telephone Interview

Task:　　　　To establish rapport with patients; to discuss provider's fees; to identify patient responsibility before the first visit.

Condition:　　Fee schedule, appointment schedule, telephone, note pad

Standards:　　Perform the Task within 15 minutes with a minimum score of _____ points.

No.	Step	Points	Check #1	Check #2	Check #3
1	Answer the phone professionally and appropriately.				
2	Demonstrate professional behavior, demeanor, and active listening skills: • Identify the caller and determine that the caller is a new patient. • Determine the nature of the appointment and suggest possible dates. • Collect the patient's basic demographic and insurance information.				
3	Explain clinic policy that copayment and coinsurance will be collected at the time of appointment.				
4	Determine if patient needs directions, and provide directions if needed. Instruct patient to arrive 15 minutes prior to appointment time.				
5	End the call professionally and appropriately. Promptly mail a Patient Information Brochure.				
Student's Total Points					
Points Possible					
Final Score (Student's Total Points/ Possible Points)					

Name _____ **Date** _____ **Score** _____

Instructor's/Evaluator's Comments and Suggestions:

_____

_____

_____

_____

_____

CHECK #1

Evaluator's Signature: _____   Date:

CHECK #2

Evaluator's Signature: _____   Date:

CHECK #3

Evaluator's Signature: _____   Date:

ABHES Competency: VI.A.1.a.2.e Use proper telephone techniques; VI.A.1.a.3.x Use physician fee schedule; VI.A.1.a.7.a Orient patients to office policies and procedures

CAAHEP Curriculum: IV.P.2 Report relevant information to others succinctly and accurately; IV.P.4 Explain general office policies; IV.P.7 Demonstrate telephone techniques

Name _____   Date _____   Score _____

COMPETENCY ASSESSMENT

Procedure 20-2   Prepare Itemized Patient Accounts for Billing in a Manual System

Task: To notify patients of the fees for services rendered and collect on those accounts.

Condition: Computer or typewriter, calculator, patient account of ledger cards, billing statement forms

Standards: Perform the Task within 20 minutes with a minimum score of _____ points.

Work Documentation: Completed patient statement

No.	Step	Points	Check #1	Check #2	Check #3
1	Gather accounts and ledgers with outstanding balances, and separate out the accounts that are overdue. Scan the accounts for possible errors.				
2	For each overdue account, create a statement which includes: • The patient's name, address, and guarantor. • Place current date on statement. Itemize the procedures in lay terms and indicate the charges for each. • Identify and subtract any payments made.The unpaid balance, totaled correctly.				
3	Discuss with the office manager the course of action to be taken on past-due accounts. If instructed, place statements in envelopes and mail.				
	Student's Total Points				
	Points Possible				
	Final Score (Student's Total Points/ Possible Points)				

Name _____ **Date** _____ **Score** _____

WORK DOCUMENTATION
*Attach completed patient statement.

Instructor's/Evaluator's Comments and Suggestions:

_____

_____

_____

_____

CHECK #1

Evaluator's Signature: _____   Date:

CHECK #2

Evaluator's Signature: _____   Date:

CHECK #3

Evaluator's Signature: _____   Date:

ABHES Competency: VI.A.1.a.3.l Perform billing and collection procedures; VI.A.1.a.8.d Manage accounts payable and receivable

CAAHEP Curriculum: VI.P.3.c Perform collections procedures

Name _____   Date _____   Score _____

COMPETENCY ASSESSMENT

Procedure 20-3   Identify Accounts Receivable Using Medical Office Simulation Software (MOSS)

Task: To determine credit balances for patient billing.

Condition: Computer, MOSS, printer

Standards: Perform the Task within 15 minutes with a minimum score of _____ points.

Work Documentation: Printed Billing and Payment report

No.	Step	Points	Check #1	Check #2	Check #3
1	Open MOSS and select Report Generation from the Main Menu.				
2	Select the "Billing and Payment Report" and print it out.				
3	Go through the printed report and correctly determine which patients have outstanding balances. Circle those patients with balances.				
4	Confirm that each patient has a balance by reviewing the patient's ledger.				
Student's Total Points					
Points Possible					
Final Score (Student's Total Points/ Possible Points)					

Name _____ Date _____ Score _____

WORK DOCUMENTATION

*Attach printed Billing and Payment report.

Instructor's/Evaluator's Comments and Suggestions:

_____

_____

_____

_____

_____

CHECK #1

Evaluator's Signature: _____ Date:

CHECK #2

Evaluator's Signature: _____ Date:

CHECK #3

Evaluator's Signature: _____ Date:

ABHES Competency: VI.A.1.a.3.d Apply computer concepts for office procedures; VI.A.1.a.3.l Perform billing and collection procedures; VI.A.1.a.8.d Manage accounts payable and receivable

CAAHEP Curriculum: VI.P.3.c Perform collections procedures; VI.P.3 Utilize computerized office billing systems

Name _____ Date _____ Score _____

COMPETENCY ASSESSMENT

Procedure 20-4 Preparing Itemized Patient Accounts for Billing Using Medical Office Simulation Software (MOSS)

Task: To notify patients of the fees for services rendered and collect on those accounts.

Condition: Computer, MOSS, Billing and Payments report generated in Procedure 20-3

Standards: Perform the Task within 15 minutes with a minimum score of _____ points.

Work Documentation: Printed Remainder Statements

No.	Step	Points	Check #1	Check #2	Check #3
1	Open MOSS and select Patient Billing from the Main Menu.				
2	Correctly populate the Patient Billing screen, selecting Remainder Statement, date range, all patients and all providers.				
3	In field 6, type "Your insurance has been billed. The balance shown is your responsibility," and in field 7, select the patients who are to receive this message.				
4	Click the Process button and review the statements on screen, comparing them with the Billing and Payment report. Print the statements.				
Student's Total Points					
Points Possible					
Final Score (Student's Total Points/ Possible Points)					

Name _____   Date _____   Score _____

WORK DOCUMENTATION

*Attached printed Remainder Statements.

Instructor's/Evaluator's Comments and Suggestions:

_____

_____

_____

_____

_____

CHECK #1

Evaluator's Signature: Date:

CHECK #2

Evaluator's Signature: Date:

CHECK #3

Evaluator's Signature: Date:

ABHES Competency: VI.A.1.a.3.d Apply computer concepts for office procedures; VI.A.1.a.3.l Perform billing and collection procedures; VI.A.1.a.8.d Manage accounts payable and receivable

CAAHEP Curriculum: VI.P.3.c Perform collections procedures; VI.P.3 Utilize computerized office billing systems

Name _____ **Date** _____ **Score** _____

COMPETENCY ASSESSMENT

Procedure 20-5   Post/Record Collection Agency Adjustments in a Manual System

Task: To keep track of financial adjustments.

Condition: Manual bookkeeping system, patient's account, black or blue and red pen for use in manual bookkeeping system

Standards: Perform the Task within 15 minutes with a minimum score of _____ points.

Work Documentation: Completed patient ledger and day sheet

No.	Step	Points	Check #1	Check #2	Check #3
1	Enter the amount received from the collection agency on the day sheet with an appropriate note in the explanation section.				
2	Record the amount received and explanation in the patient's account. Subtract the amount received from the patient's account balance, and place this remainder value in the adjustment column.				
3	Subtract the amount paid by the collection agency from the patient's account. Write off the amount that is not collectable.				
4	Correctly enter the difference between the amount collected and the amount paid by the collection agency (plus the agency's fee) as a negative adjustment.				
	Student's Total Points				
	Points Possible				
	Final Score (Student's Total Points/ Possible Points)				

Name _____ **Date** _____ **Score** _____

WORK DOCUMENTATION
*Attach completed patient ledger and day sheet.

_____

Instructor's/Evaluator's Comments and Suggestions:

_____

_____

_____

_____

_____

CHECK #1

Evaluator's Signature: _____   Date:

CHECK #2

Evaluator's Signature: _____   Date:

CHECK #3

Evaluator's Signature: _____   Date:

ABHES Competency: VI.A.1.a.3.s Post collection agency payments; VI.A.1.a.8.d Manage accounts payable and receivable

CAAHEP Curriculum: VI.P.2.a Post entries on a day sheet; VI.P.2.h Post collection agency payments

Name _____   Date _____   Score _____

COMPETENCY ASSESSMENT

Procedure 20-6   Post/Record Adjustments Using Medical Office Simulation Software (MOSS)

Task: To keep track of financial adjustments.

Condition: Computer, MOSS, Post/Record Adjustments Exercises in Procedure 20-6

Standards: Perform the Task within 15 minutes with a minimum score of _____ points.

Work
Documentation: Screen shot of the completed Payment Posting screen

No.	Step	Points	Check #1	Check #2	Check #3
1	Open MOSS and select Payment Posting from the Main Menu.				
2	Find Megan Caldwell in the patient menu and select Apply Payment. Correctly Post the adjustment to her account (take a screen shot of the completed screen after the adjustment has been entered). Close out of patient account.				
3	Find Justin McNamara in the patient menu and select Apply Payment. Correctly Post the adjustment to his account (take a screen shot of the completed screen after the adjustment has been entered). Close out of patient account.				
4	Find Evan Lagasse in the patient menu and select Apply Payment. Correctly Post the adjustment to his account (take a screen shot of the completed screen after the adjustment has been entered). Close out of patient account.				
Student's Total Points					
Points Possible					
Final Score (Student's Total Points/ Possible Points)					

Name _____   **Date** _____   **Score** _____

WORK DOCUMENTATION

*Attach screen shot of the completed Payment Posting screens.

_____

Instructor's/Evaluator's Comments and Suggestions:

_____

_____

_____

_____

_____

CHECK #1

Evaluator's Signature: _____   Date:

CHECK #2

Evaluator's Signature: _____   Date:

CHECK #3

Evaluator's Signature: _____   Date:

ABHES Competency: VI.A.1.a.3.d Apply computer concepts for office procedures; VI.A.1.a.3.o Post adjustments

CAAHEP Curriculum: VI.P.2.d Post adjustments; VI.P.3 Utilize computerized office billing systems

Name _____   Date _____   Score _____

COMPETENCY ASSESSMENT

Procedure 21-1   Preparing Accounts Receivable Trial Balance in a Manual System

Task: A trial balance will determine if there is any problem between the daily journal and the ledger or patient accounts.

Condition: Patient accounts, calculator

Standards: Perform the Task within 20 minutes with a minimum score of _____ points.

Work Documentation: Correct totals in Work Documentation section

No.	Step	Points	Check #1	Check #2	Check #3
1	Pull all patient accounts that have a balance due.				
2	Correctly add all balances together.				
3	Correctly determine the accounts receivable total: A. Enter the accounts receivable total. B. Add total charges for this month. Subtotal. C. Subtract the total payments from B. D. Total the amount of the month's adjustments. Subtract this number from C.				
4	The calculations in steps 2 and 3 match (the outstanding patient accounts and the accounts receivable total).				
Student's Total Points					
Points Possible					
Final Score (Student's Total Points/ Possible Points)					

Name _____ **Date** _____ **Score** _____

WORK DOCUMENTATION

Total of Patient Ledgers that have balances: _____

Accounts receivable total:

    A. Monthly accounts receivable total: _____

    B. Add total of this month's charges: + _____

                     Subtotal: _____

    C. Subtract total payments: − _____

                     Subtotal: _____

    D. Total of the month's adjustments: _____

        Subtract D from C for TOTAL: _____

Instructor's/Evaluator's Comments and Suggestions:

_____

_____

_____

_____

_____

CHECK #1

Evaluator's Signature: _____ Date:

CHECK #2

Evaluator's Signature: _____ Date:

CHECK #3

Evaluator's Signature: _____ Date:

ABHES Competency: VI.A.1.a.8.d Manage accounts payable and receivable

Name _____ **Date** _____ **Score** _____

COMPETENCY ASSESSMENT

Procedure 21-2   Preparing Accounts Receivable Trial Balance Using Medical Office Simulation Software (MOSS)

Task: A trial balance will determine if there is any problem between the daily journal and the ledger or patient accounts.

Condition: Computer, MOSS, printer

Standards: Perform the Task within 15 minutes with a minimum score of _____ points.

Work Documentation: Printed Monthly Summary report

No.	Step	Points	Check #1	Check #2	Check #3
1	Open MOSS and select Report Generation from the Main Menu.				
2	Select the "Monthly Summary." Review the report for errors.				
3	Print the report.				
	Student's Total Points				
	Points Possible				
	Final Score (Student's Total Points/ Possible Points)				

Name _____ **Date** _____ **Score** _____

WORK DOCUMENTATION
*Attach printed Monthly Summary report.

_____

Instructor's/Evaluator's Comments and Suggestions:

_____

_____

_____

_____

_____

CHECK #1	
Evaluator's Signature:	Date:

CHECK #2	
Evaluator's Signature:	Date:

CHECK #3	
Evaluator's Signature:	Date:

ABHES Competency: VI.A.1.a.3.d Apply computer concepts for office procedures; VI.A.1.a.8.d Manage accounts payable and receivable

CAAHEP Curriculum: VI.P.3 Utilize computerized office billing systems

Name _____   **Date** _____   **Score** _____

COMPETENCY ASSESSMENT

Procedure 22-1   Completing a Medical Incident Report

Task: To complete a medical incident report and submit it in a timely manner.

Condition: Appropriate medical incident report form or computer with Incident Report Software

Standards: Perform the Task within 15 minutes with a minimum score of _____ points.

Work
Documentation: Completed incident report form

No.	Step	Points	Check #1	Check #2	Check #3
1	Accurately completed the incident report form, filling in each section of the report, including: • Used quotes when referring to un-witnessed statements. • Wrote the names of all witnesses to the incident in the report.				
2	Submitted the completed incident report to the appropriate person.				
Student's Total Points					
Points Possible					
Final Score (Student's Total Points/ Possible Points)					

Name _____ Date _____ Score _____

WORK DOCUMENTATION
*Attach completed incident report form.

_____

Instructor's/Evaluator's Comments and Suggestions:

_____
_____
_____
_____
_____

CHECK #1

Evaluator's Signature: _____ Date: _____

CHECK #2

Evaluator's Signature: _____ Date: _____

CHECK #3

Evaluator's Signature: _____ Date: _____

ABHES Competency: VI.A.1.a.5.h Perform risk management procedures

CAAHEP Curriculum: IX.P.6 Complete an incident report

Name _____ **Date** _____ **Score** _____

COMPETENCY ASSESSMENT

Procedure 22-2   Preparing a Meeting Agenda

Task: To prepare a meeting agenda with an established list of specific items to be discussed or acted on, or both.

Condition: List of participants, the order of business, names of individuals giving reports, names of any guest speakers, a computer, paper on which to print agendas

Standards: Perform the Task within 20 minutes with a minimum score of _____ points.

Work Documentation: Printed agenda

No.	Step	Points	Check #1	Check #2	Check #3
1	Confirmed the proposed dates and place of meeting.				
2	Prepared and typed agenda: • Collected information from previous meetings' minutes for old agenda items. • Checked with others for report items and determined any new business.				
3	When completed, had agenda approved by the meeting chair.				
4	Sent agenda to participants.				
5	Reserved meeting room and arranged for food items, equipment, and supplies that may be needed.				
Student's Total Points					
Points Possible					
Final Score (Student's Total Points/ Possible Points)					

Name _____ **Date** _____ **Score** _____

WORK DOCUMENTATION

*Attach printed agenda.

_____

Instructor's/Evaluator's Comments and Suggestions:

_____
_____
_____
_____
_____

CHECK #1	
Evaluator's Signature:	Date:

CHECK #2	
Evaluator's Signature:	Date:

CHECK #3	
Evaluator's Signature:	Date:

ABHES Competency: VI.A.1.a.2.j Use correct grammar, spelling and formatting techniques in written works; VI.A.1.a.2.o Fundamental writing skills; VI.A.1.a.3.a Perform basic secretarial skills

CAAHEP Curriculum: IV.P.2 Report relevant information to others succinctly and accurately

Name _____   **Date** _____   **Score** _____

COMPETENCY ASSESSMENT

Procedure 22-3   Supervising a Student Practicum

Task: To prepare a training path for a student extern being assigned to the office, make the involved personnel aware of their responsibilities, preplan the jobs the student will perform and in what sequence they will be assigned, and try to make the externship successful by providing as much supervision and assistance as necessary.

Condition: A schedule log, calendar, office procedures manual, any criteria presented by the program director

Standards: Perform the Task within 30 minutes with a minimum score of _____ points.

No.	Step	Points	Check #1	Check #2	Check #3
1	Reviewed the clinical practicum contract between your agency and the educational institution.				
2	Identified student's supervisor, planned tasks that the student will perform, and created a schedule for the student and staff.				
3	Oriented the student to the facility and staff upon arrival.				
4	Maintained an accurate record of hours the student worked, including missed days and late arrivals.				
5	Consulted with providers, staff, and the student for feedback.				
6	Reported student progress to the medical assistants program director and prepared student's evaluation report using input from all who worked with student.				
Student's Total Points					
Points Possible					
Final Score (Student's Total Points/ Possible Points)					

Name _____   **Date** _____   **Score** _____

Instructor's/Evaluator's Comments and Suggestions:

_____

_____

_____

_____

_____

CHECK #1

Evaluator's Signature: _____   Date:

CHECK #2

Evaluator's Signature: _____   Date:

CHECK #3

Evaluator's Signature: _____   Date:

ABHES Competency: VI.A.1.a.2.m Adaptation for individualized needs; VI.A.1.a.7.d orient and train personnel

CAAHEP Curriculum: IV.P.4 Explain general office policies

Name _____ **Date** _____ **Score** _____

COMPETENCY ASSESSMENT

Procedure 22-4   Developing and Maintaining a Procedure Manual

Task: To develop and maintain a comprehensive, up-to-date procedures manual covering each medical, technical, and administrative procedure in the office with step-by-step directions and rationale for performing each task.

Condition: A computer, three-ring binder, paper, procedures, and criteria

Standards: Perform the Task within 20 minutes with a minimum score of _____ points.

Work Documentation: Binder with procedure entries

No.	Step	Points	Check #1	Check #2	Check #3
1	Wrote detailed, step-by-step procedures and rationale for each medical, technical, and administrative function. Each procedure was written by experienced employees close to the function and reviewed by a supervisor or the office manager.				
2	Included regular maintenance (cleaning, servicing, and calibrating) instructions and flow sheets for all office equipment, both in the clinical area and in the office/business areas.				
3	Included step-by-step procedures on how to accomplish each task, both in the clinical area and in the office/business areas.				
4	Included local and out of the area resources for clinical staff, office/business staff, physicians/providers, and patients. Provided a listing in each area with contact information and services available.				
5	Included basic rules and regulations, state and federal, which are related to processes performed in both clinical and office/business areas.				
6	Included the clinic procedures and flow sheets for taking inventory in each of the areas, and instructions on ordering procedures.				
7	Collected the procedures into the office procedures manual.				
Student's Total Points					
Points Possible					
Final Score (Student's Total Points/ Possible Points)					

Name _____   Date _____   Score _____

WORK DOCUMENTATION
*Attach completed procedure manual entries.

_____

Instructor's/Evaluator's Comments and Suggestions:

_____

_____

_____

_____

_____

CHECK #1

Evaluator's Signature: Date:

CHECK #2

Evaluator's Signature: Date:

CHECK #3

Evaluator's Signature: Date:

ABHES Competency: VI.A.1.a.6.a Maintain physical plant; VI.A.1.a.7.d Orient and train personnel

CAAHEP Curriculum: IX.P.5 Incorporate the Patient's Bill of Rights into personal practice and medical office policies and procedures; IX.P.8 Apply local, state and federal health care legislation and regulation appropriate to the medical assisting practice setting

Name _____ **Date** _____ **Score** _____

COMPETENCY ASSESSMENT

Procedure 22-5 Making Travel Arrangements with a Travel Agent

Task: To make travel arrangements for the provider.

Condition: A travel plan/preferences, telephone, directory, computer, and the provider's or office credit card to secure reservations

Standards: Perform the Task within 20 minutes with a minimum score of _____ points.

Work Documentation: Completed itinerary

No.	Step	Points	Check #1	Check #2	Check #3
1	Confirmed the details of the trip: dates, times, places of departures and arrivals, preferred transportation method, number of travelers, preferred lodging type, and price range.				
2	Telephoned travel agent.				
3	Picked up tickets or arranged for delivery or secured confirmation of electronic tickets. Checked that flight, rental car, room arrangements were accurate and confirmed.				
4	Made copies of itinerary, forwarded one to the provider and maintained one copy in the office.				
Student's Total Points					
Points Possible					
Final Score (Student's Total Points/ Possible Points)					

Name _____   **Date** _____   **Score** _____

WORK DOCUMENTATION

*Attach completed itinerary.

Instructor's/Evaluator's Comments and Suggestions:

_____

_____

_____

_____

_____

CHECK #1

Evaluator's Signature: Date:

CHECK #2

Evaluator's Signature: Date:

CHECK #3

Evaluator's Signature: Date:

ABHES Competency: VI.A.1.a.3.f Manage physician's professional schedule and travel

Name _____ **Date** _____ **Score** _____

COMPETENCY ASSESSMENT

Procedure 22-6   Making Travel Arrangements via the Internet

Task: To make travel arrangements for the provider using the Internet.

Condition: A travel plan/preferences, computer, and the provider's or office credit card to secure reservations

Standards: Perform the Task within 20 minutes with a minimum score of _____ points.

Work Documentation: Completed itinerary

No.	Step	Points	Check #1	Check #2	Check #3
1	Confirmed the details of the trip: dates, times, places of departures and arrivals, preferred transportation method, number of travelers, preferred lodging type, and price range.				
2	Made arrangements using the Internet.				
3	Picked up tickets or arranged for delivery or secured confirmation of electronic tickets. Checked that flight, rental car, room arrangements were accurate and confirmed.				
4	Made copies of itinerary, forwarded one to the provider and maintained one copy in the office.				
Student's Total Points					
Points Possible					
Final Score (Student's Total Points/ Possible Points)					

Name _____   **Date** _____   **Score** _____

WORK DOCUMENTATION

*Attach completed itinerary.

_____

Instructor's/Evaluator's Comments and Suggestions:

_____

_____

_____

_____

_____

CHECK #1

Evaluator's Signature: _____   Date: _____

CHECK #2

Evaluator's Signature: _____   Date: _____

CHECK #3

Evaluator's Signature: _____   Date: _____

ABHES Competency: VI.A.1.a.3.f Manage physician's professional schedule and travel

CAAHEP Curriculum: V.P.7 Use internet to access information related to the medical office

Name _____   **Date** _____   **Score** _____

COMPETENCY ASSESSMENT

Procedure 22-7   Processing Employee Payroll

Task:　　　　To process payroll compensating employees, calculating all deductions accurately.

Condition:　 Computer and payroll software or checkbook; tax withholding tables; Federal Employers Tax Guide

Standards:　 Perform the Task within 45 minutes with a minimum score of _____ points.

No.	Step	Points	Check #1	Check #2	Check #3
1	Reviewed time cards and determined each employee's time away from the office.				
2	Calculated the salary or hourly wages owed to each employee; calculated the deductions that must be withheld form the paycheck for each employee.				
3	Used computer and payroll software or handwrote the payroll checks for each employee, with explanation of deductions.				
4	Mailed each payroll check to the appropriate employee.				
Student's Total Points					
Points Possible					
Final Score (Student's Total Points/ Possible Points)					

Name _____ **Date** _____ **Score** _____

Instructor's/Evaluator's Comments and Suggestions:

_____

_____

_____

_____

_____

CHECK #1

Evaluator's Signature: _____ Date:

CHECK #2

Evaluator's Signature: _____ Date:

CHECK #3

Evaluator's Signature: _____ Date:

ABHES Competency: VI.A.1.a.8.f Process employee payroll

Name _____   **Date** _____   **Score** _____

COMPETENCY ASSESSMENT

Procedure 22-8   Perform an Inventory of Equipment and Supplies

Task: To develop an inventory of expendable administrative and clinical supplies in a medical office.

Condition: Printout of most recent inventory spreadsheet, clipboard, pad of reorder forms, pen or pencil

Standards: Perform the Task within 15 minutes with a minimum score of _____ points.

Work Documentation: Completed inventory list

No.	Step	Points	Check #1	Check #2	Check #3
1	Assembled equipment and supplies to be inventoried.				
2	Accurately counted and recorded the quantity of each item and completed an inventory form.				
3	If a supply or equipment was below the minimum amount, indicated that reordering was necessary.				
4	Signed form and gave to person responsible for ordering supplies. Or filled out an order form for the additional supplies.				
Student's Total Points					
Points Possible					
Final Score (Student's Total Points/ Possible Points)					

Name _____ **Date** _____ **Score** _____

WORK DOCUMENTATION

*Attach completed inventory list.

_____

Instructor's/Evaluator's Comments and Suggestions:

_____

_____

_____

_____

_____

CHECK #1

Evaluator's Signature: _____ Date:

CHECK #2

Evaluator's Signature: _____ Date:

CHECK #3

Evaluator's Signature: _____ Date:

ABHES Competency: VI.A.1.a.6.c Inventory equipment and supplies; VI.A.1.a.6.d Evaluate and recommend equipment and supplies for practice

CAAHEP Curriculum: V.P.10 Perform an office inventory

Name _____ **Date** _____ **Score** _____

COMPETENCY ASSESSMENT

Procedure 22-9 Perform Routine Maintenance or Calibration of Administrative and Clinical Equipment

Task: To ensure the operability and calibration of administrative and clinical equipment.

Condition: Equipment list with maintenance or calibration requirements; clipboard, pen, maintenance record sheets, and deficiency tags; access to operation and service manuals of equipment to be serviced; access to any necessary maintenance tools and supplies

Standards: Perform the Task within 30 minutes with a minimum score of _____ points.

Work Documentation: Maintenance record form

No.	Step	Points	Check #1	Check #2	Check #3
1	Inspected appropriate administrative and clinical equipment. Inspected for cleanliness, safety, and operability. Noted and recorded equipment that required repairs.				
2	Properly completed maintenance checklist: • Included date. • Documented whether maintenance or repairs were needed. • Signed the form.				
	Student's Total Points				
	Points Possible				
	Final Score (Student's Total Points/ Possible Points)				

Name _____ **Date** _____ **Score** _____

WORK DOCUMENTATION

*Attach maintenance record form.

Instructor's/Evaluator's Comments and Suggestions:

_____

_____

_____

_____

_____

CHECK #1

Evaluator's Signature: _____ Date: _____

CHECK #2

Evaluator's Signature: _____ Date: _____

CHECK #3

Evaluator's Signature: _____ Date: _____

ABHES Competency: VI.A.1.a.6.b Operate and maintain facilities and perform routine maintenance of administrative and clinical equipment safely

CAAHEP Curriculum: V.P.9 Perform routine maintenance of office equipment with documentation

Name _____   **Date** _____   **Score** _____

COMPETENCY ASSESSMENT

Procedure 23-1   Develop and Maintain a Policy Manual

Task: To develop and maintain a comprehensive, up-to-date policy manual of all office policies relating to employee practices, benefits, office conduct, and so forth.

Condition: Computer, three-ring binder, paper, standard policy format

Standards: Perform the Task within 20 minutes with a minimum score of _____ points.

Work
Documentation: Printed policy manual entries

No.	Step	Points	Check #1	Check #2	Check #3
1	Following office format, developed precise, written office policies detailing all necessary information pertaining to the staff and their positions. Included benefits, vacation, sick leave, hours, dress codes, evaluations, rules of conduct, and grounds for dismissal.				
2	Identified procedures for reimbursing overtime, preventing discrimination and harassment, creating a safe workplace, and allowing for jury duty.				
3	Included a policy statement related to smoking and other substances.				
4	Identified steps to follow should an employee become disabled during employment.				
5	Determined what employee opportunities for continuing education would be reimbursed and included requirements for certification and licensures.				
6	Provided a copy of the policy manual for each employee.				
7	Reviewed and updated the policy manual regularly. Added or deleted items as necessary, dating each revision.				
Student's Total Points					
Points Possible					
Final Score (Student's Total Points/ Possible Points)					

Name _____ **Date** _____ **Score** _____

WORK DOCUMENTATION

*Attach printed policy manual entries.

Instructor's/Evaluator's Comments and Suggestions:

_____
_____
_____
_____
_____

CHECK #1
Evaluator's Signature: Date:

CHECK #2
Evaluator's Signature: Date:

CHECK #3
Evaluator's Signature: Date:

ABHES Competency: VI.A.1.a.7.d Orient and train personnel

CAAHEP Curriculum: IV.P.4 Explain general office policies

Name _____ **Date** _____ **Score** _____

COMPETENCY ASSESSMENT

Procedure 23-2   Prepare a Job Description

Task: To develop a precise definition of the tasks assigned to a job, to determine the expectations and level of competency required, and to specify the experience, training, and education needed to perform the job for purposes of recruiting and performance evaluation.

Condition: Computer, three-ring binder, paper, standard job description format

Standards: Perform the Task within 20 minutes with a minimum score of _____ points.

Work Documentation: Printout of job description, or job description written in documentation area

No.	Step	Points	Check #1	Check #2	Check #3
1	Detailed each task that creates the job.				
2	Listed special medical, technical, or clerical skills needed.				
3	Determined the level of education, training, and experience required for the position.				
4	Determined where the job fits into the overall structure of the office.				
5	Specified any unusual working conditions (hours, locations, etc.) that may apply.				
6	Described career path opportunities.				
7	Reviewed and updated the policy manual regularly. Added or deleted items as necessary, dating each revision.				
Student's Total Points					
Points Possible					
Final Score (Student's Total Points/ Possible Points)					

Name _____ **Date** _____ **Score** _____

WORK DOCUMENTATION

Instructor's/Evaluator's Comments and Suggestions:

_____
_____
_____
_____
_____

CHECK #1

Evaluator's Signature: Date:

CHECK #2

Evaluator's Signature: Date:

CHECK #3

Evaluator's Signature: Date:

ABHES Competency: VI.A.1.a.6.a Maintain physical plant

CAAHEP Curriculum: IV.P.4 Explain general office policies

Name _____ **Date** _____ **Score** _____

COMPETENCY ASSESSMENT

Procedure 23-3   Conduct Interviews

Task: To screen applicants for training, experience, and characteristics to select the best candidate to fill the position vacancy.

Condition: Interview questions; policy manual (for referencing); applicant's résumé, application, and cover letter

Standards: Perform the Task within 40 minutes with a minimum score of _____ points.

No.	Step	Points	Check #1	Check #2	Check #3
1	Reviewed résumés and applications received and selected candidates who had the skills being sought. Created an interview worksheet for each candidate, listing the points to cover, and identified who on staff would be part of the interview team.				
2	Screened the applicant over the phone.				
3	Conducted the in-office interview of the applicant: • Provided an overview about the practice and staff, describing the job and answering preliminary questions. • Asked questions about the applicant's work experience and educational background. • Informed the applicants when a decision would be made, and thanked each applicant for participating in the interview.				
4	Checked references of all prospective employees.				
5	Established a second interview for the qualified candidate if necessary.				
6	Confirmed accepted job offers in writing, specifying the details of the offer and acceptance, and notified all unsuccessful applicants by letter when the position was filled.				
	Student's Total Points				
	Points Possible				
	Final Score (Student's Total Points/ Possible Points)				

Name _____ **Date** _____ **Score** _____

Instructor's/Evaluator's Comments and Suggestions:

_____

_____

_____

_____

_____

CHECK #1	
Evaluator's Signature:	Date:

CHECK #2	
Evaluator's Signature:	Date:

CHECK #3	
Evaluator's Signature:	Date:

ABHES Competency: VI.A.1.a.2.f Interview effectively; VI.A.1.a.2.i Recognize and respond to verbal and non-verbal communication; VI.A.1.a.2.k Principles of verbal and nonverbal communication; VI.A.1.a.2.l Recognition and response to verbal and non-verbal communication

CAAHEP Curriculum: IV.P.2 Report relevant information to others succinctly and accurately; IV.P.4 Explain general office policies

Name _____   **Date** _____   **Score** _____

COMPETENCY ASSESSMENT

Procedure 23-4   Orient Personnel

Task: To acquaint new employees with office policies, staff, what the job encompasses, procedures to be performed, and job performance expectations.

Condition: Policy manual

Standards: Perform the Task within 30 minutes with a minimum score of _____ points.

No.	Step	Points	Check #1	Check #2	Check #3
1	Toured the facilities and introduced the office staff. Assigned a mentor from the staff to help with the orientation.				
2	Completed employee-related documents and explained their purpose. Explained the benefits program.				
3	Presented the office policy manual and discussed the key elements. Reviewed federal and state regulatory precautions for medical facilities. Reviewed the job description.				
4	Explained and demonstrated procedures to be performed and the use of procedures manuals supporting these procedures.				
5	Demonstrated the use of any specialized equipment (such as time clocks, key entries, etc.). Medical equipment would be demonstrated by clinical staff.				
	Student's Total Points				
	Points Possible				
	Final Score (Student's Total Points/ Possible Points)				

Name _____   **Date** _____   **Score** _____

Instructor's/Evaluator's Comments and Suggestions:

_____

_____

_____

_____

_____

CHECK #1

Evaluator's Signature: _____   Date: _____

CHECK #2

Evaluator's Signature: _____   Date: _____

CHECK #3

Evaluator's Signature: _____   Date: _____

ABHES Competency: VI.A.1.a.7.d Orient and train personnel

CAAHEP Curriculum: IV.P.4 Explain general office policies

Comprehensive Examination

1. Which term describes false and malicious writing about another that constitutes defamation of character?

    a. Slander

    b. Assault

    c. Libel

    d. Invasion of privacy

    e. Battery

2. When reviewing a résumé, the human resources manager does NOT consider the applicant's:

    a. supplemental education

    b. unexplained gaps in employment

    c. training related to the position

    d. age, sex, and race

    e. previous experience

3. The standard of professional conduct for a certified medical assistant should be:

    a. in keeping with the AAMA Code of Ethics

    b. outlined by the provider or employer

    c. based on the Hippocratic oath

    d. in keeping with the AMA Principles of Medical Ethics

    e. determined by the state's medical practice act

4. After an interview, the applicant should:

    a. telephone to say thank you

    b. have his or her references call the interviewer

    c. telephone after three days to check the status of his or her application

    d. promptly send a follow-up letter

    e. send a lavish thank-you gift

5. A medical assistant must NEVER:

    a. perform a venipuncture

    b. perform a laboratory test

    c. imply that he or she is a nurse

    d. dispense a medication after a direct order from the provider

    e. give a medication after a direct order from the provider

6. Which legal principle is violated when a medical assistant practices outside of his or her training?

    a. Public d'uty

    b. Consent

    c. Privacy rights

    d. Confidentiality

    e. Standard of care

7. Which manner of dress is appropriate for an interview?

   a. A medical assistant's uniform

   b. Evening makeup

   c. Spectacular nail polish

   d. Casual clothing

   e. Neat business attire

8. Which statement accurately describes ethics?

   a. Ethics are a personal moral philosophy of right and wrong.

   b. Ethics are a code of minimal acceptable behavior.

   c. Ethics are the state's legal standards established for a profession.

   d. Ethics are the federal legal standards established for a profession.

   e. Ethics are standards for personal behavior as established by organized religions.

9. When stressed, we may exhibit all of the following EXCEPT:

   a. anxiety

   b. objective thinking

   c. depression

   d. anger

   e. irrational behavior

10. All of the following statements about Good Samaritan laws are true EXCEPT:

    a. These laws do not provide legal protection to on-duty emergency care providers.

    b. Providers must act in a reasonable and prudent manner.

    c. The conditions of these laws vary in each state.

    d. No matter what their level of training, providers must do everything for the patient.

    e. Health care providers are ethically, not legally, obligated to assist in emergency situations.

11. What is the purpose of the certification credential for medical assistants?

    a. The certification credential is required for graduation.

    b. The certification credential guarantees a job.

    c. The certification credential meets state registration requirements.

    d. The certification credential indicates a medical assistant's professional and technical competence.

    e. The certification credential meets state licensure requirements.

12. Consent for treatment may usually be given by:

    a. the patient's closest relative

    b. a patient in a mental institution

    c. any minor over 16

    d. the person accompanying the patient

    e. a legally competent patient

13. Who is the most important member of the health care team?

    a. The patient

    b. The provider

    c. The medical assistant

    d. The nurse

    e. The receptionist

14. All of the following cultural influences may affect communication EXCEPT:

    a. education

    b. sexual orientation

    c. ethnic heritage

    d. geographic location

    e. age

15. When the medical office wins in small claims court, the money is collected from the patient by:

    a. the bailiff

    b. the patient's insurance company

    c. the probate court

    d. the medical office

    e. the court-appointed collection agency

16. Which statement is accurate regarding the Americans with Disabilities Act (ADA)?

    a. The ADA applies only to medical practices and health care facilities.

    b. The ADA applies to all businesses.

    c. The ADA applies only to businesses with 15 or more employees.

    d. The ADA applies only to businesses with 50 or more employees.

    e. The ADA applies only to state and federal government agencies.

17. Which governmental agency requires employers to ensure employee safety concerning occupational exposure to potentially harmful substances?

    a. CDC

    b. HCFA

    c. OSHA

    d. USPS

    e. Department of Health and Human Services

18. The certifying board of which organization awards the CMA credential?

    a. AAMA

    b. AMT

    c. ABHES

    d. CAAHEP

    e. RMA

19. The certifying board of which organization awards the RMA credential?

    a. AAMA

    b. ABHES

    c. CAAHEP

    d. CMA

    e. AMT

20. Which of the following might be expected as an Asian expression of pain?

    a. Descriptive words such as "piercing" or "throbbing"

    b. A description of disturbances of the mind

    c. Ranking pain on a scale of 1 to 10

    d. Moaning and crying out

    e. Descriptive terms of body imbalance

21. How often must the CMA (AAMA) credential be renewed?

    a. Annually

    b. Every five years

    c. Biannually

    d. Every three years

    e. With every job change

22. What is the highest level in Maslow's hierarchy of needs?

    a. Safety needs

    b. Love needs

    c. Self-actualization

    d. Belongingness needs

    e. Esteem needs

23. Which of the following information is considered to be public domain?

    a. A person's sexual preference

    b. A person's police record

    c. A person's past drug addiction

    d. A person's HIV-positive status

    e. A person's alcoholism

24. The goal of the National Health Information Network is to create a:

    a. unified EMR for all health care facilities

    b. standard for computer hardware in health care facilities

    c. support network for health care facilities transitioning to EMR

    d. method of communicating EMR software program options

    e. system for exchange of health care information

25. Dr. Bennett's office will be switching to an EMR system. The office manager communicates to staff that they will be using a "remote hosted" system. This means that:

    a. the software will be run from a server in the office, which requires the purchase of only one software license

    b. the software will be installed on each individual computer, and each individual computer will require its own license

    c. the software is owned and maintained by another company, but the office will pay for the right to log in and use the system

    d. a software company will log in to the office computers in order to install and maintain the software

    e. the system will require the use of very complex hardware and additional training for staff

26. An individual who has done something that results in damage to another person or his or her property would be prosecuted under what type of law?

    a. Statute

    b. Case

    c. Breach of contract

    d. Tort

    e. Regulatory

27. Which of the following would NOT be considered an intentional tort?

    a. Defamation of character

    b. Invasion of privacy

    c. Assault

    d. Negligence

    e. Fraud

28. A patient who is undergoing a surgical procedure signs a consent for treatment. The consent would be referred to as a(n):

    a. expressed contract

    b. implied contract

    c. breach of contract

    d. tort contract

    e. consideration contract

29. Licensing for health care professionals, health department regulations, and regulations for mandatory reporting are all examples of:

    a. civil law

    b. administrative law

    c. criminal law

    d. negligent law

    e. contract law

30. A durable power of attorney document indicates:

    a. what type of medical treatment a patient wishes to have during end-of-life care

    b. who the patient would like to make decisions for him if he cannot make decisions himself

    c. what (if any) organs a patient would like to donate

    d. Do Not Resuscitate orders

    e. consent for surgical treatment

31. A medical professional who is convicted of nonfeasance would have:

    a. performed a treatment improperly

    b. performed an illegal act

    c. failed to perform necessary treatment

    d. violated confidentiality

    e. performed a duty outside of her scope of practice

32. Statutes of limitation apply to everything but:

    a. negligence

    b. fraud

    c. malfeasance

    d. dereliction of duty

    e. murder

33. Health care workers are mandatory reporters in all BUT which of the following situations?

    a. Child abuse

    b. Elder abuse

    c. Alcoholism

    d. Communicable diseases

    e. Death

34. Which of the following is true of HIPAA?

    a. Hospitals are prevented from releasing homicide or other crime-related information to law enforcement agencies.

    b. Students performing internships may not have access to computer systems in health care facilities.

    c. The HIPAA prevents health care facilities from sharing information with health care providers who are not their employees even when the information is essential for patient treatment.

    d. Health care facilities should appoint a privacy officer and adopt procedures for handling requests.

    e. HIPAA regulations do not apply to patients seeking care under government assistance programs.

35. The stage of grief in which patients attempt to make promises in order to change their situation would be considered:

    a. denial

    b. bargaining

    c. anger

    d. depression

    e. acceptance

36. End-of-life palliative care is most often provided by:

    a. hospice

    b. acute care hospitals

    c. rehabilitation hospitals

    d. skilled nursing facilities

    e. assisted living facilities

37. The AAMA code of ethics for medical assistants includes statements about each of the following EXCEPT:

    a. honor

    b. confidentiality

    c. continuing education

    d. improving community

    e. supervising provider

38. A medical office that transmits information over a wireless network must ensure that:

    a. the network allows staff to transmit information from home

    b. the network allows the provider to transmit information while doing patient visits at the hospital

    c. each staff member understands the encryption of the network

    d. the network meets HIPAA guidelines

    e. the network can be accessed by the appropriate insurance companies

39. Advanced Beneficiary Notices must be used for patients with what type of insurance?

    a. Medicaid

    b. Workers Compensation

    c. Medicare

    d. Blue Cross/Blue Shield

    e. TRICARE

40. Which of the following helps a medical assistant to manage time well?

    a. Reading email while answering patient calls

    b. Asking patients to jot down their complaints in their charts

    c. Asking patients to email rather than call with questions

    d. Asking front office staff to obtain patients' complaint

    e. Identifying priorities

41. Which of the following is NOT an important quality for a medical assistant?

    a. Ability to manage time efficiently

    b. Ability to delegate

    c. Initiative

    d. Flexibility

    e. Ability to work as a team member

42. Which of the following is an important aspect of verbal communication?

    a. Facial expressions

    b. Appearance

    c. Tone of voice

    d. Body language

    e. Gestures

43. The most important component of the message you communicate is:

    a. Perception of the person receiving the message

    b. Tone of voice

    c. The vocabulary used

    d. Facial expression

    e. Body language

44. Nancy, the medical assistant you work with, always changes the subject when you bring up topics that she does not want to discuss. This behavior would be considered:

    a. assertive

    b. passive

    c. aggressive

    d. professional

    e. passive-aggressive

45. Which of the following is NOT considered a part of negligence?

    a. Duty

    b. Dereliction

    c. Denial

    d. Direct cause

    e. Damages

46. The "base" of a medical word is called the:

    a. prefix

    b. suffix

    c. combining form

    d. root

    e. anatomical

47. The provider you are working with asks you to place a bandage just proximal to the knee. You would place the bandage:

    a. just below the knee

    b. on the front of the knee

    c. on the back of the knee

    d. just above the knee

    e. covering the entire knee area from top to bottom

48. You read a medical report that indicates that a provider made an incision from the superior to the inferior portion of the heart during a surgery. This means that the incision was made in the:

   a. frontal plane

   b. coronal plane

   c. transverse plane

   d. superior plane

   e. horizontal plane

49. The sac that covers the heart is referred to as the:

   a. pericardium

   b. epicardium

   c. endocardium

   d. myocardium

   e. mediastinum

50. The structure that is responsible for the formation of urine is the:

   a. medulla

   b. cortex

   c. nephron

   d. major calyx

   e. minor calyx

51. The congenital disorder that involves one or more vertebrae that do not close is called:

   a. cerebral palsy

   b. muscular dystrophy

   c. Tay-Sachs disease

   d. spina bifida

   e. hydrocele

52. Which of the following is a characteristic of a malignant tumor?

   a. Smooth borders

   b. Irregular shape

   c. Slow growth

   d. Well-differentiated cells

   e. Encapsulation

53. Muscular movements that are out of conscious control (e.g., the heart beating) are called:

   a. voluntary

   b. involuntary

   c. agonist

   d. antagonist

   e. synergistic

54. The type of joint that allows for the greatest range of motion is the:

    a. hinge

    b. suture

    c. pivot

    d. cartilaginous

    e. ball and socket

55. The portion of the brain that is responsible for higher thought processes such as logical thinking is the:

    a. parietal lobe

    b. frontal lobe

    c. occipital lobe

    d. temporal lobe

    e. cerebellum

56. An individual with a blood type of O positive is considered:

    a. a universal recipient

    b. ineligible to donate

    c. able to donate only to people with O positive blood

    d. able to donate only to people with only O negative blood

    e. a universal donor

57. The type of immunity that is developed from being vaccinated is:

    a. naturally acquired active immunity

    b. artificially acquired passive immunity

    c. artificially acquired active immunity

    d. naturally acquired passive immunity

    e. naturally acquired active passive immunity

58. An X-ray that is shot from the back of the person toward the front would be considered:

    a. AP

    b. lateral

    c. oblique

    d. PA

    e. transverse

59. Which of the following is NOT a portion of the large intestine?

    a. Duodenum

    b. Cecum

    c. Transverse colon

    d. Rectum

    e. Ascending colon

60. When performing screening, the medical assistant must:

    a. diagnose patients' symptoms

    b. prioritize patients' needs

    c. allow patients to determine their own needs

    d. schedule patients in the order in which they arrive

    e. evaluate patients' ability to pay

61. A person with a hypersensitivity to a bee sting may go into:

    a. cardiac arrest

    b. neurogenic shock

    c. anaphylactic shock

    d. seizures

    e. respiratory shock

62. All of the following statements about shock are accurate EXCEPT:

    a. There is inadequate circulation to body parts.

    b. The patient's body is kept warm to prevent chilling.

    c. The patient's pulse becomes rapid and weak.

    d. The medical assistant can administer medication as ordered by the provider.

    e. The patient's blood pressure increases.

63. Which of the following is a major disadvantage of NOT seeking care for an illness until it becomes very advanced?

    a. The patient does not have time to deal with death.

    b. Pain management and treatment may not work as well as they could have.

    c. The family can prepare without frightening the patient.

    d. Denial postpones the inevitable.

    e. The patient does not have time to create advance directives.

64. Redirecting a socially unacceptable impulse into one that is socially acceptable is called:

    a. regression

    b. repression

    c. projection

    d. sublimation

    e. denial

65. You are a medical assistant in an ambulatory care facility, and an emergency situation arises. What should you do first?

    a. Notify the provider.

    b. Give first aid.

    c. Assess the patient.

    d. Call 911.

    e. Evaluate the causes.

66. The act of evaluating the urgency of a medical situation and prioritizing treatment is known as:

    a. screening

    b. empathy

    c. trauma

    d. diagnosing

    e. sorting

67. Which condition is detected with the Mantoux test?

    a. HIV

    b. Syphilis

    c. PKU

    d. TB

    e. Infectious mononucleosis

68. Which of the following is used as a contrast medium for a radiographic lower GI examination?

    a. Air

    b. Iodine salts

    c. Water

    d. A barium swallow

    e. A barium enema

69. Which type of pathogen causes mumps, measles, and chicken pox?

    a. Bacteria

    b. Viruses

    c. Spirochetes

    d. Parasites

    e. Rickettsiae

70. Which body system does the acronym PERRLA refer to?

    a. Cardiovascular system

    b. Gastrointestinal system

    c. Nervous system

    d. Respiratory system

    e. Urogenital system

71. Which term means difficulty breathing?

    a. Apnea

    b. Bradypnea

    c. Tachypnea

    d. Eupnea

    e. Dyspnea

72. Which of the following statements is accurate regarding vitamins?

    a. Vitamins A, B, D, and E are fat soluble.

    b. Vitamins are needed in large quantities.

    c. Water-soluble vitamins are stored in fatty tissues.

    d. Vitamins are simple molecules.

    e. Vitamins B and C are water soluble.

73. Which statement is accurate regarding ventricular tachycardia?

    a. Ventricular tachycardia causes severe chest pain.

    b. Ventricular tachycardia is life threatening.

    c. Ventricular tachycardia is often seen in patients using depressants.

    d. Ventricular tachycardia has a cardiac cycle that occurs early.

    e. Ventricular tachycardia occurs in healthy people.

74. Which genetic disorder is characterized by mental retardation?

    a. Sickle cell anemia

    b. Huntington's disease

    c. Down's syndrome

    d. Cystic fibrosis

    e. Pernicious anemia

75. Which type of nutrient contains the most calories per gram?

    a. Carbohydrate

    b. Protein

    c. Mineral

    d. Fat

    e. Vitamin

76. Which term describes a reason why a medication should NOT be administered?

    a. Side effect

    b. Contraindication

    c. Potentiation

    d. Idiosyncratic

    e. Cross-tolerance

77. Robby is coming down with chicken pox but does not have any symptoms yet. He is now at the:

    a. acute stage

    b. convalescent stage

    c. declining stage

    d. incubation stage

    e. prodromal stage

78. Which of the following statements about medical asepsis hand washing is accurate?

    a. Medical assistants should turn the faucet on with a clean, dry paper towel.

    b. Medical assistants should hold their hands upward.

    c. Medical assistants should scrub up to their elbows.

    d. Medical assistants should touch only the inside of the sink with their hands.

    e. Medical assistants should turn off the faucet with a used paper towel.

79. Which of these positions is used for the treatment and examination of the back and buttocks?

    a. Trendelenburg

    b. Dorsal recumbent

    c. Lithotomy

    d. Supine

    e. Prone

80. Which term describes a woman who has never been pregnant?

    a. Multigravida

    b. Nullipara

    c. Nulligravida

    d. Multipara

    e. Primipara

81. Which infection control guidelines are used by all health care professionals for all patients?

    a. Body Substance Isolation guidelines

    b. Standard Precautions

    c. OSHA guidelines

    d. Transmission-Based Precautions

    e. Universal Precautions

82. All of the following are acceptable wrappings for autoclaving EXCEPT:

    a. plastic pouches

    b. muslin

    c. paper bags

    d. aluminum foil

    e. paper wrapping

83. The most common disorder of the urinary system is:

    a. renal calculi

    b. urinary tract infection

    c. glomerulonephritis

    d. cystitis

    e. pyelonephritis

84. Which of the following diseases is sexually transmitted?

    a. Pelvic inflammatory disease

    b. Cervical cancer

    c. Endometriosis

    d. Prostatitis

    e. Ovarian cancer

85. Which term describes an infection of the middle ear?

    a. Otitis externa

    b. Otalgia

    c. Otitis media

    d. Otorrhagia

    e. Otosclerosis

86. Which condition is commonly known as fainting?

    a. Tinnitus

    b. Singultus

    c. Bruit

    d. Syncope

    e. Vertigo

87. Which of the following is a progressive degenerative disease of the liver?

    a. Hepatitis A

    b. Cholecystitis

    c. Hepatomegaly

    d. Hepatitis B

    e. Cirrhosis

88. Which type of injection is made into the fatty layer just below the skin?

    a. Intramuscular

    b. Subcutaneous

    c. Intradermal

    d. Intravenous

    e. Intermuscular

89. An elevation of which blood cell count indicates the presence of inflammation in the body?

    a. Platelet count

    b. Erythrocyte sedimentation rate

    c. Hematocrit

    d. Total hemoglobin

    e. White blood cell differentiation

90. What condition is characterized by an abnormal thickening and hardening of the skin?

    a. Acne

    b. Melanoma

    c. Dermatophytosis

    d. Scleroderma

    e. Psoriasis

91. Who discovered penicillin?

    a. Sir Alexander Fleming

    b. Robert Koch

    c. Louis Pasteur

    d. Joseph Lister

    e. Edward Jenner

92. Homeostasis refers to what?

    a. A sterile environment

    b. A complete procedure

    c. Everyone getting along

    d. Internal equilibrium

    e. Rapid heart rate

93. The classification of drugs with the lowest potential of abuse is:

    a. Schedule IV

    b. Schedule I

    c. Schedule V

    d. Schedule II

    e. Schedule III

94. The provider you are working with asks you to provide a patient with samples of a new medication. By doing so, you are:

    a. prescribing medication

    b. administering medication

    c. compounding medication

    d. mixing medication

    e. dispensing medication

95. Which of the following is information about a medication that is NOT found in the PDR?

    a. Indications for use

    b. The shape of each pill

    c. Dosage and administration route

    d. Precautions

    e. Generic name

96. A drug that increases the effect of another has which type of effect?

    a. Local

    b. Remote

    c. Synergistic

    d. Systemic

    e. Topical

97. A medication that is ordered to be delivered in a sublingual route would be:

    a. placed in the cheek

    b. swallowed

    c. inserted into the rectum

    d. placed under the tongue

    e. placed on top of the tongue

98. A medication that is classified as an expectorant would have what effect?

    a. Dilate bronchi

    b. Prevent coughing

    c. Relax blood vessels

    d. Decrease nausea

    e. Increase the amount of mucus being expelled

99. A medication that increases the amount of urine excreted by the body would be classified as a(n):

    a. diuretic

    b. antiarrhythmic

    c. antiemetic

    d. vasopressor

    e. muscle relaxant

100. All of the following are part of a medication order EXCEPT:

    a. name of drug

    b. who dispenses the medication

    c. form of drug

    d. route of administration

    e. prescribing provider's signature

101. A prescription that indicates a medication should be administered "OD" would go where?

    a. Left eye

    b. Right ear

    c. Left ear

    d. Right eye

    e. In the nose

102. The metric prefix which refers to one-millionth of a unit is:

    a. milli

    b. kilo

    c. meter

    d. gram

    e. micro

103. Pediatric medication dosages are figured based on the child's:

    a. height

    b. age

    c. weight

    d. gender

    e. chest circumference

104. A patient weighs 130 pounds. The provider asked you to convert that weight into kilograms. You know that there are 2.2 pounds in 1 kilogram. How many kilograms does this patient weigh?

    a. 4.55 kg

    b. 59.09 kg

    c. 286 kg

    d. .07 kg

    e. 260 kg

105. Which of the following is NOT 1 of the 6 rights?

    a. Dose

    b. Provider

    c. Route

    d. Patient

    e. Drug

106. Parenteral medication is administered via:

    a. the mouth

    b. the rectum

    c. the skin

    d. inhalation

    e. an injection

107. The type of injection that is administered at a 90-degree angle is:

    a. subcutaneous

    b. intradermal

    c. intravenous

    d. inhaled

    e. intramuscular

108. Hypodermic needles are most appropriate for what?

    a. Venipuncture

    b. Aspirations

    c. Allergy injections

    d. Intramuscular and subcutaneous injections

    e. Insulin administration

109. Which of the following is NOT an appropriate injection site for an intramuscular injection?

    a. Dorsogluteal

    b. Biceps

    c. Ventrogluteal

    d. Deltoid

    e. Vastus lateralis

110. Which of the following points is the highest point in a normal ECG graph?

    a. P

    b. Q

    c. R

    d. S

    e. T

111. The yellow portion of the safety warning label indicates which of the following?

    a. Chemical instability

    b. Health hazard

    c. Fire hazard

    d. PPE requirements

    e. Biohazard level

112. A chemical that is extremely flammable would be given a safety rating of:

    a. 3

    b. 2

    c. 1

    d. 4

    e. 0

113. The component of blood that is responsible for clotting is:

    a. Erythrocyte

    b. Leukocyte

    c. Plasma

    d. Serum

    e. Thrombocyte

114. Which of the following substances is NOT a normal component of urine?

    a. Ammonia

    b. Blood

    c. Creatinine

    d. Urea

    e. Water

115. The type of urine sample that requires a patient to avoid eating and drinking prior to voiding is:

    a. 24-hour

    b. first-morning

    c. fasting

    d. random

    e. catheter collection

116. Which of the following is NOT a component of the physical examination of urine?

    a. Volume

    b. Color

    c. Unusual

    d. Specific gravity

    e. pH

117. Casts found in urine are formed from:

    a. carbohydrates

    b. lipids

    c. calcium

    d. proteins

    e. potassium

118. Exposing bacterial growth to an antibiotic in order to determine effective treatment of an infection is called:

    a. culturing

    b. taxonomy

    c. sensitivity testing

    d. inoculation

    e. Gram stain

119. The disease of the eye that is characterized by an elevated intraocular pressure is:

    a. cataract

    b. glaucoma

    c. macular degeneration

    d. amblyopia

    e. strabismus

120. The mineral that is important for the formation of bone tissue is:

    a. calcium

    b. potassium

    c. zinc

    d. iron

    e. magnesium

121. Which of the following is a type of bacteria?

    a. Streptococci

    b. Helminth

    c. Protozoa

    d. Tinea

    e. Scabies

122. Diseases caused by which type of pathogen are treated by antibiotics?

    a. Protozoa

    b. Fungi

    c. Bacteria

    d. Virus

    e. Parasite

123. Personal protective equipment should always be used in each of the follow situations EXCEPT:

    a. handling processing a urine specimen

    b. taking vital signs

    c. performing venipuncture

    d. assisting with surgical procedures

    e. disinfecting instruments

124. A worker who is exposed to bodily fluids through an accidental needlestick from a contaminated needle should immediately flush the area with:

    a. alcohol

    b. hydrogen peroxide

    c. betadine

    d. bleach

    e. water

125. Which immunization must be available free to all health care employees?

    a. Hepatitis A

    b. Hepatitis C

    c. Hepatitis B

    d. HIV

    e. TB

126. Use of alcohol-based hand rub is acceptable in which of the following situations?

    a. Before and after eating

    b. Before and after using the restroom

    c. After contact with body excretions

    d. After decontamination of a work area

    e. Following processing of microbiological specimens

127. Which of the following is NOT an OSHA requirement for housekeeping in a medical setting?

    a. Routine decontamination of reusable containers

    b. Double-bagged soiled linens

    c. Biohazard waste collected in impermeable red containers

    d. Sharps containers stored in an upright condition

    e. Alcohol-based hand rub available at all times

128. When performing CPR on an infant or child, circulation is checked by assessing pulse at which pulse point?

    a. Carotid

    b. Axial

    c. Femoral

    d. Brachial

    e. Dorsal pedis

129. The method used to clear an airway obstruction in an unconscious adult is:

    a. finger sweep

    b. back blows

    c. chest thrust

    d. 2 rescue breaths

    e. CPR

130. A burn that has penetrated to the bone would be considered:

    a. superficial

    b. partial thickness

    c. 100%

    d. full thickness

    e. 75%

131. Which of the following is NOT a step in controlling bleeding from an open wound on the arm?

    a. Applying direct pressure

    b. Elevating the arm

    c. Wrapping the wound tightly

    d. Applying pressure to the appropriate artery

    e. Disinfecting the area

132. Appropriate first aid for a patient with a case of acute frostbite would include:

    a. immersing the area in warm water

    b. warming the area by creating friction

    c. immediately raising the patient's core body temperature

    d. applying heavy moisturizing cream to the area

    e. immediately debriding necrotic tissues

133. Appropriate treatment for an acute sprain or strain would include all BUT which of the following?

    a. Ice

    b. Rest

    c. Compression

    d. Range of motion

    e. Elevation

134. A medication that is to be taken twice a day would be indicated as:

    a. qd

    b. tid

    c. qid

    d. bid

    e. od

135. Which type of manual identifies the specific methods for performing tasks?

    a. Policy

    b. Training

    c. Procedures

    d. Personnel

    e. Benefits

136. What is the primary purpose of managed care plans?

    a. To allow patients to manage their own care

    b. To control patients' access to providers

    c. To encourage patients to explore alternative medicine treatments

    d. To provide acute care only

    e. To provide comprehensive health care at a reasonable cost

137. How are claims managed when both parents are covered by health insurance?

    a. The father's plan is always primary.

    b. Claims for the family are paid according to the birthday rule.

    c. The mother's plan is always primary.

    d. Double benefits are paid for the children.

    e. The duplication of benefits rule is put into effect.

138. Why are accurate medical records legally important?

    a. Because they are needed to provide referrals

    b. Because they assist in controlling health care costs

    c. Because they aid in billing

    d. Because they are written documentation used to prove patient care

    e. Because they are essential to quality patient care

139. Which type of check is used most often for writing payroll checks?

    a. Voucher check

    b. Traveler's check

    c. Certified check

    d. Cashier's check

    e. Money order

140. What is the role of a computer firewall?

    a. A computer firewall limits potential damage from viruses.

    b. A computer firewall protects the computer in the event of a fire.

    c. A computer firewall does not allow outside computers access to your computer.

    d. A computer firewall allows outside access to an office computer but not to databases.

    e. A computer firewall prevents employees from surfing the Internet for personal reasons.

141. How should a letter that requires a written receipt be mailed?

    a. Registered mail

    b. Priority mail

    c. Third-class mail

    d. Certified mail

    e. First-class mail

142. Which of the following are used in conjunction with CPT codes?

    a. V Codes

    b. Preventive care codes

    c. Injury codes

    d. Modifiers

    e. E Codes

143. What must happen when more than one policy pays on a claim?

    a. Coinsurance

    b. Coordination of benefits

    c. Co-pay

    d. Deductible

    e. Exclusions

144. When alphabetizing and assigning units for filing order, titles are considered:

    a. as part of the last name

    b. as the first indexing unit

    c. as the third indexing unit

    d. as part of the patient's surname

    e. as a separate unit at the end

145. A person who is injured on the job may be covered by:

    a. workers' compensation

    b. CHAMPUS

    c. Medicaid

    d. disability insurance

    e. HCFA

146. Which of the following is an advantage of accepting credit cards in an ambulatory care setting?

    a. Maintaining patient confidentiality is not a problem.

    b. There are no fees to be paid by the practice.

    c. The money is available to the practice within one day.

    d. The money is usually available to the practice within 10 days.

    e. Accepting credit cards eliminates having to file insurance claims.

147. What is the key to having an effective scheduling system?

    a. Accommodating patient preferences

    b. Customizing the system to the type of practice

    c. Tailoring the system to provider preferences

    d. Accommodating the requirements of the insurance carriers

    e. Effectively monitoring the use of time versus the dollars produced

148. Which scheduling system assigns two patients to the same time?

    a. Clustering

    b. Stream

    c. Modified wave

    d. Double booking

    e. Open-hours

149. Which program provides health care coverage for low-income individuals?

    a. CHAMPUS

    b. Workers' compensation

    c. Medicare

    d. CHAMPVA

    e. Medicaid

150. Which of the following is a critical issue regarding the use of a fax machine in a medical office?

    a. The speed at which the machine works

    b. The time required to train personnel

    c. Compromised confidentiality due to access by unauthorized personnel

    d. The clarity of the documents received

    e. The volume of documents the machine can handle

151. Which of the following is used when there is not enough information to find a more specific code?

    a. NEC

    b. NOS

    c. CC

    d. V Codes

    e. E Codes

152. Which of the following tells the computer hardware what to do?

    a. Application software

    b. The motherboard

    c. The modem

    d. System software

    e. Servers

153. Which of the following conditions is most frequently related to the repetitive use of a computer?

    a. Eyestrain

    b. Fatigue

    c. Carpal tunnel syndrome

    d. Lower back pain

    e. Tension headaches

154. When seeking employment, a person who has job experience should use:

    a. a targeted résumé

    b. a functional résumé

    c. a complete résumé

    d. an Information Mapping résumé

    e. a chronological résumé

155. Which type of résumé highlights one's special qualities?

    a. Targeted

    b. Functional

    c. Chronological

    d. Concise

    e. Career oriented

156. Which statement is accurate regarding a cover letter?

    a. The cover letter may be addressed "To whom it may concern."

    b. The purpose of the cover letter is to ask for an interview.

    c. The cover letter includes résumé information.

    d. The cover letter should be bulleted.

    e. The cover letter should include a list of references.

157. Which of the following tasks is NOT assigned to the human resources manager?

    a. Creating office manuals

    b. Hiring and firing personnel

    c. Interpreting legal regulations

    d. Providing employee training

    e. Performing employee evaluations

158. Tiffany wants a well-paying position as a medical assistant. Which statement is accurate regarding her search?

    a. Every CMA (AAMA) is guaranteed a well-paying position.

    b. Using an employment agency is her most effective tool in finding a well-paying position.

    c. Networking is her most effective tool in finding a well-paying position.

    d. Running down all leads is her most effective tool in finding a well-paying position.

    e. Cold calling to offices that are not advertising will produce excellent leads.

159. Which federal law requires employers to verify the right of employees to work in the United States?

    a. Immigration Reform Act

    b. Equal Pay Act

    c. Civil Rights Act

    d. Fair Labor Standards Act

    e. Americans with Disabilities Act

160. Which of these interviewing tips is accurate?

    a. Think carefully before answering questions.

    b. Do not ask questions, as you may appear confused.

    c. Answer questions "off the cuff" so your responses do not seem rehearsed.

    d. Place your personal belongings—coat, purse, and so on—on the interviewer's desk.

    e. Give lengthy answers to all questions, even when you are not sure of the answer.

161. Which of the following statements about completing an employment application form is accurate?

    a. Write "See résumé" rather than repeating information.

    b. Using either a pen or pencil is acceptable.

    c. Try to complete the application without referring to your résumé.

    d. Complete the application quickly to demonstrate how well you work.

    e. Following instructions is very important.

162. Which of the following is the best networking resource for recruiting new personnel?

    a. Newspapers

    b. Family and friends

    c. Current employees

    d. Patients

    e. AAMA's national office

163. All of these interview questions are appropriate EXCEPT:

    a. "What is most important to you about this job?"

    b. "What is your clinical experience?"

    c. "Have you ever been bonded before?"

    d. "Do you have any health-related problems that might affect your job performance?"

    e. "Where did you go to school?"

164. Which of the following is NOT vital résumé information?

    a. Home address

    b. Current telephone number

    c. Education

    d. Date of birth

    e. Work experience

165. Which payroll forms must be submitted to the Social Security Administration each year?

    a. W-4

    b. W-2

    c. W-6

    d. 1099

    e. 941

166. A policy manual should include all of the following EXCEPT:

    a. employment practices

    b. insurance billing techniques

    c. wage and salary scales

    d. evaluation schedules

    e. continuing education policies

167. In order to track inventory in an office, the most appropriate type of software to use would be:

    a. word processing

    b. billing

    c. contact management

    d. spreadsheet

    e. EMR

168. When taking a telephone message, everything BUT the following should be included:

    a. full name of person leaving message

    b. reason for the call

    c. time and date of call

    d. expected action

    e. diagnosis of the patient the message is about

169. An office operating on a wave schedule will:

    a. have groups of patients arriving at relatively the same time throughout the day

    b. schedule two patients for the same appointment time

    c. schedule patients in specific time increments (e.g., every 15 minutes)

    d. allow for walk-in patients at any time

    e. provide "catch up" time for the provider

170. When scheduling an outpatient procedure, each of the following should be completed EXCEPT:

    a. obtaining necessary preauthorizations

    b. making arrangements with the facility

    c. notifying the patient of the arrangements

    d. determining and scheduling preprocedure testing

    e. precertifying the admission

171. A block letter style includes:

    a. centered paragraphs with all other components at the left margin

    b. all components starting at the left margin

    c. centered address and signature lines with paragraphs starting at the left margin

    d. centered address, signature line, and first paragraph

    e. all components centered

172. Source-oriented medical records are organized by the:

    a. cause of a patient's medical diagnosis

    b. location of a patient's medical record

    c. nature of a patient's complaint

    d. treatment methods being used

    e. professionals who have documented in the record

173. Each of the following is objective information EXCEPT:

    a. laboratory data

    b. diagnosis

    c. prescribed treatment

    d. patient's complaint

    e. exam findings

174. Color coding medical records assists with each of the following EXCEPT:

    a. increasing efficiency with filing

    b. increasing the ability to identify filing errors

    c. identifying a patient's diagnosis

    d. identifying patients who are due for a physical during a specific month

    e. removing inactive files

175. Tickler files are helpful in:

    a. sending billing notices

    b. scheduling the provider's time

    c. providing reminders for routine medical appointments

    d. submitting insurance claims

    e. processing payroll

176. Providers' fees are generally set by each of the following EXCEPT:

    a. reasonable

    b. insurance

    c. customary

    d. usual

    e. geographic region

177. Accounts receivable refers to:

    a. money collected by a practice during a day

    b. accounts turned over to a debt collection agency

    c. money owed by the practice

    d. money owed to a practice

    e. petty cash expenditures

178. Manually posting charges usually involves each of the following EXCEPT:

    a. day sheet

    b. ledger card

    c. account summary

    d. encounter form

    e. HCFA 1500

179. The Truth in Lending Act requires:

    a. lower interest rates for medical services

    b. an increased amount of time for repayment of medical loans

    c. use of an independent billing service

    d. accurate information regarding finance charges

    e. routine billing statements

180. Calls made to a patient's home in order to collect money owed to a practice are regulated by:

    a. the Truth in Lending Act

    b. CLIA

    c. the Fair Debt Collection Act

    d. OSHA

    e. AMA

181. Once an account has been submitted to a collection agency, the medical assistant should:

    a. discontinue sending statements to the patient

    b. continue to send routine billing statements to the patient

    c. send copies of billing statements to emergency contacts listed in the patient's chart

    d. file for legal action in small claims court

    e. telephone the patient in order to attempt to collect the debt

182. Best practices with manual bookkeeping involve all of the following EXCEPT:

    a. proficiency with 10-key typing

    b. using consistent methods

    c. writing with red ink

    d. writing numbers clearly

    e. double checking all math

183. In managing practice finances, an adjustment would be used for:

    a. recording payment

    b. recording charges

    c. indicating past due accounts

    d. indicating discounts or write-offs

    e. indicating accounts turned over to collections

184. When preparing a check to a supplier, the medical assistant should:

    a. verify the expense has been approved

    b. endorse with "for deposit only"

    c. reconcile the bank statement

    d. record the payment on the correct ledger card

    e. file a I-9 tax form

185. If an office determines it will accept personal checks as payment, it is important to:

    a. clearly post the policy

    b. implement use of a restrictive endorsement

    c. follow Truth in Lending guidelines

    d. verify policies with the practice's bank

    e. follow Fair Debt collection guidelines

186. Mrs. Jones's insurance requires that she pay for $400 of medical expenses before she is eligible for insurance payment for medical services. The $400 would be referred to as:

    a. a co-payment

    b. coinsurance

    c. a deductible

    d. a premium

    e. an exclusion

187. Mr. Johnson's insurance company has stated that it will not pay for treatment of his asthma because he was known to have the disease prior to the time when his policy was purchased. His asthma would be considered a(n):

    a. exclusion

    b. preexisting condition

    c. concurrent condition

    d. secondary diagnosis

    e. subjective condition

188. The type of Medicare coverage that provides benefits for inpatient medical care is:

    a. Medicare B

    b. Medicare D

    c. Medicare E

    d. Medicare A

    e. Medicare F

189. Most managed care organizations provide a capitated payment for services. This means that:

    a. a maximum payment for services is set

    b. patients must pay excess charges out of their own pocket

    c. they will not pay for services covered by another company

    d. the government sets the maximum allowed charge for a service

    e. patients' premiums will never change

190. RBRVS payment structures are based on all EXCEPT which of the following?

    a. Level of work

    b. Malpractice expenses

    c. Regional charges

    d. Diagnosis of patient

    e. Experience of the provider

191. E Codes in the ICD book are used to identify:

    a. wellness-related procedures

    b. cardiovascular diseases

    c. morphology

    d. neurological diseases

    e. accidents

192. V Codes in the ICD book are used to identify:

    a. accidents

    b. cardiovascular disease

    c. wellness-related procedures

    d. morphology

    e. neurological diseases

193. Which of the following would be considered a commercial form of health insurance?

    a. Medicare

    b. Medicaid

    c. CHAMPUS

    d. Blue Cross/Blue Shield

    e. Workers compensation

194. Patient Sally Kane arrives at your office as a new patient. While copying her insurance card you notice that she will need to pay 20 percent of the cost of the visit. That percentage is referred to as:

    a. co-payment

    b. coinsurance

    c. deductible

    d. premium

    e. exclusion

195. In order to accurately locate an ICD code, which section of the book would you use first?

    a. Volume II

    b. Volume I

    c. Volume III

    d. Volume IV

    e. Appendix

196. Which of the following is NOT a section in the CPT book?

    a. Anesthesia

    b. Surgery

    c. Pathology and Laboratory

    d. Rehabilitation

    e. Medicine

197. Deliberately billing a service at a higher level than what was completed would be considered:

    a. downcoding

    b. bundling

    c. unbundling

    d. upcoding

    e. proper procedure

198. A business letter sent from an office would be processed through which class of mail?

    a. Second class

    b. Third class

    c. First class

    d. Fourth class

    e. Priority mail

199. Hospital inpatient payments are based on:

    a. APG

    b. DRG

    c. Usual fees

    d. Reasonable fees

    e. Customary fees

200. Dr. Abernathy provides you with the growth chart appearing on the following page and asks you to explain it to the child's mother, who is concerned that the child is not as tall as other children his age. You would explain to the mother that:

    a. the child is actually slightly above average on the growth chart

    b. the child is actually slightly below average on the growth chart

    c. the child is actually well above average on the growth chart

    d. the child is actually well below average on the growth chart

    e. the child is of average height on the growth chart

CDC Growth Charts: United States

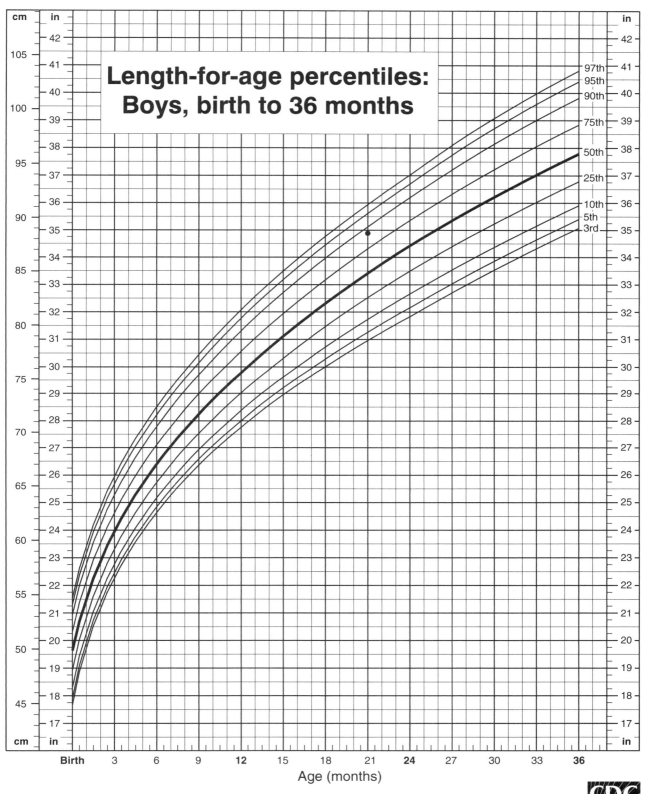

Length-for-age percentiles: Boys, birth to 36 months

Age (months)

Published May 30, 2000.
SOURCE: Developed by the National Center for Health Statistics in collaboration with
the National Center for Chronic Disease Prevention and Health Promotion (2000).

CDC

SAFER · HEALTHIER · PEOPLE™